$TO

AN EX-SMOKER'S SURVIVAL GUIDE

POSITIVE STEPS TO A SLIM, TRANQUIL, SMOKE-FREE LIFE

–by–

**Lesley Sussman &
Sally Bordwell**

McGraw-Hill Book Company

*New York   St. Louis   San Francisco   Bogotá
Guatemala   Hamburg   Lisbon   Madrid
Mexico   Montreal   Panama   Paris   San Juan
São Paulo   Tokyo   Toronto*

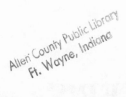

1 2 3 4 5 6 7 8 9   FGRFGR   8 7 6

ISBN 0-07-062344-9

LIBRARY OF CONGRESS CATALOGING-IN-PUBLICATION DATA

Sussman, Lesley 1944–
  An ex-smoker's guide to survival.
  Bibliography: p.
  Includes index.
  1. Tobacco habit—Prevention.   2. Behavioral modification.   I. Bordwell, Sally, 1947–   II. Title.
RC567.S85   1986   616.86′505   86–2846
ISBN 0–07–062344–9

MRP Design.

Breathing exercises from Philip Smith's book, *Total Breathing*, used with the permission of the McGraw-Hill Book Company.

Breathing exercises from *Breathing: The ABC's*, by Carola H. Speads used with permission of the author.

Information on beginning a self-help group used with permission of the New York City Self-Help Clearinghouse and the National Self-Help Clearinghouse.

Portions of *Exercise Equivalents of Foods: A Practical Guide for the Overweight*, by Frank Konishi used with permission of Southern Illinois University Press.

The 14-day quit-smoking plan used with permission of the American Lung Association.

*To the courageous men and women
everywhere who are determined not
to let their lives go up in smoke.*

2289815

CONTENTS

CONTENTS

FOREWORD

This is a book I wish had been available to me when I quit smoking three years ago. If it had been, it might have lessened—perhaps even prevented—some of the turmoil I went through as a result of giving up cigarettes.

Frankly, those hours, days—even weeks—after I put out my last cigarette were among the toughest in my life. Not only did I have to muster every ounce of willpower to keep from rushing out to the nearest store and purchasing a pack of cigarettes, but I also found myself gaining weight no matter how hard I tried not to.

I began to feel cheated by all those quit-smoking programs which promised to help me make the transition so effortlessly from being almost a pack-and-a-half-a-day smoker to a non-smoker, but failed to do so.

I also grew angry at my family and friends whose congratulations that I had stopped smoking turned into admonishments that I was eating too much—especially when I knew that I was reducing my normal intake of food.

At first only a few additional pounds registered on the bathroom scale, causing me to joke that my jeans were getting too tight. I began experimenting with strange combinations of low-calorie meals, and prowled supermarket aisles for diet products. But after only two months of not smoking, I had put on fifteen pounds and could no longer even fit into my jeans!

What was happening to me? I just couldn't understand it. Was I the only ex-smoker to be so afflicted? Gaining pounds was bad enough, but I was also experiencing a general feeling of depression. It was only much later that I learned that these doldrums are nicotine-induced, and are fairly common to almost anyone who gives up cigarettes. But because I didn't realize this at the time, I began seeing a therapist in search of clues to my bummed-out state of mind.

It was on a sweltering July afternoon, when I had just returned from my therapist's office where I once again threatened to resume smoking, that I met a long-time friend—Les Sussman—for a drink at a neighborhood café.

I poured out my liturgy of frustrations to him, which prompted a reply that perhaps there were some books available that dealt with the trials and tribulations of new ex-smokers.

We decided to inquire at a few local bookstores and, much to our dismay, found no book which explored in any great detail such postquitting syndromes. Now even more curious, we paid a visit to the University of Illinois Medical Center Library and began to peruse research journals.

The remarkable array of current research material we discovered astounded us. Why wasn't this vital information being passed on to the millions of people who each year give up cigarettes or seriously plan to? We clearly saw the task which lay before us, and you are now reading the results of our efforts.

It was on January 26, 1983, that I smoked my last cigarette—a date that is indelibly etched in my mind. I did not realize then that I was about to embark on one of the most remarkable journeys of my life—one that led me from hypnotists to therapists and even, at times, threatened my relationship with my family and friends.

Ultimately, however, that experience resulted in a happy ending—a smoke-free me and the writing of this book. So, if you are about to embark on your own journey to a smoke-free you, begin the voyage with the knowledge that the goal is really worth it.

And remember to keep this book handy. Let it serve you as your guide should you encounter any obstacles in your efforts to remain smokeless. Above all, always remember: Don't look back!

—SALLY BORDWELL

ACKNOWLEDGMENTS

A great deal of professional assistance and encouragement was rendered to us during the difficult months of researching and writing this book. First of all, we would like to give special thanks to Dr. Frederick Bordwell, Ph.D., of the Northwestern University School of Chemistry, for reviewing much of the scientific data. Also greatly appreciated is the assistance and encouragement given us by Dr. Ned Dikmen, Ph.D. Most of our research was conducted at the University of Illinois Medical Center Library, and we cannot give enough thanks to the enthusiastic staff who helped guide us through the maze of technical journals to be found there. A special debt of gratitude to Steve Guback, director of information for the President's Council on Physical Fitness and Sports. Also thanks to the nice people at the New York City Self-Help Clearinghouse, the New York City Bureau of Nutrition, the American Dietetic

Association, and Marjorie Molyneaux of the Illinois Interagency Council on Smoking and Disease. Also aiding our efforts were the Chicago Heart Association, the American Cancer Society and its Los Angeles component, Celebrities Against Cancer, the American Lung Association, and the staffs of the Chicago Public Library and the Oak Park, Illinois, Public Library. And, finally, this book would not be possible without the strong support of our hard-nosed editor, Mrs. Lou Ashworth, and our persistent agent and good friend, Mrs. Bobbe Siegel.

PREFACE

- Does the brain contain a mysterious chemical which may cause you to want to smoke?
- Is there a substance manufactured by the body that can ease the debilitating effects of nicotine withdrawal?
- Are you aware that quitting smoking can cause depression and other negative emotions? What causes such mood swings and can anything be done to counter these feelings?
- Why is exercise one of the keys to remaining smoke-less?
- Why is nicotine the weight-conscious ex-smoker's worst enemy?
- Did you know that smokers actually eat more food than nonsmokers but still remain thinner?

These and many other often surprising, little-known facts about giving up cigarettes are revealed in this book, which takes a unique approach to an age-old problem.

If you have just quit smoking, or seriously intend to do so, *An Ex-Smoker's Survival Guide* is must reading. After all, your survival as a nonsmoker is at stake here!

The reason for writing this book was quite a simple one, and the answer often surprises people. It was written because no other book quite like it has been done before. It certainly surprised us to learn that, although there were many books in print on the subject of *how* to quit smoking, there was not one comprehensive work on how to remain smoke-free once you quit the habit. Thus we strongly believed that there was a vital need for a book of this type.

Smoking is clearly the largest preventable cause of illness and premature death in the United States. Despite the best efforts of the tobacco industry to convince us otherwise, the message must have somehow gotten through to the public because studies indicate that an astonishing 85 percent of smokers would like to stop smoking.

Each year some 2 million people do give up cigarettes. Unfortunately, only about 25 percent of smokers who do quit remain smokeless. This is the first book to explore many of the reasons why the recidivism rate is so high. It was in search of answers to this problem that we first began our research, combing through hundreds of scientific studies on the subject of smoking cessation and other related areas.

One explanation, we discovered, is that new ex-smokers are likely to suffer a variety of physical and psychological reactions when they quit smoking, and many of these reactions often make it difficult not to reach for a cigarette. Many of these changes are linked to the sudden absence of nicotine in the bloodstream.

Another important disclosure discussed in this book focuses on recent evidence that some cigarette users may actually be *physically* as well as psychologically addicted to smoking—a little-known discovery which shatters traditional beliefs that all it takes is an act of willpower to stay off cigarettes.

Ex-smokers who read this book will also learn that such feelings as depression or anger may have a physical basis caused by nicotine withdrawal. Furthermore, they will be introduced to new scientific research which can effectively help the new nonsmoker to combat such mood swings.

Predictably, our research found that some new ex-smokers gain weight. *An Ex-Smoker's Survival Guide* not only discusses the reasons why some former smokers find themselves putting on pounds, but extensively discusses ways to reverse this situation. You will even find a section containing low-calorie recipes to assist you in the battle of the bulge.

Finally, we examine smoking cessation in the light of long-term behavioral change. We discuss at length what positive steps new ex-smokers should take to help insure their success in remaining smoke-free as well as in other areas of their life.

Throughout this book we have always kept in mind the simple axiom that all of us are individuals. There are no two people, smokers, or former smokers who are exactly alike. Therefore we have offered a variety of approaches toward remaining smokeless, so that readers may tailor a program best suited to their own individual needs. This applies whether we are discussing weight gain, stress, or exercise. Use whatever works best for you.

You will be learning a lot about yourself by the time you're through reading this book—why you smoke, what's behind that sudden weight gain or those uncharacteristic mood swings, and much, much more.

Most importantly, you will learn what practical and easy-to-understand steps can be taken to cope with the negative effects of nicotine withdrawal. You will also be exposed to the latest scientific research on the effects of nicotine addiction—much of this material never before made readily available to the general public.

By the time you complete this book, you will be armed with survival techniques to help you cope with most of the problems you may encounter once you quit smoking. Again, adapt any or all of these techniques to fit your own special needs.

That's what survival and this book are all about . . . adaptation, endurance, perseverance, and, above all, a positive mental attitude.

* * *

"I felt that cancer and its possible consequence was not a suitable alternative for living, so I quit smoking. This may all sound very dull save one thing, the fantastic desire to live. Nothing so stupid as a cigarette will keep me from that."

—*NANCY WALKER*
(from a letter to the authors)

AN
EX-SMOKER'S
SURVIVAL
GUIDE

A SPECIAL INTRODUCTION: FOR SMOKERS ONLY

If you've finally smoked your last cigarette, congratulations! You've joined a growing number of Americans who each year also decide to quit the habit. As a new ex-smoker, there is no need to read this chapter, so proceed to Chapter 1.

On the other hand, if you haven't quite managed to snuff out that last cigarette yet, then this introduction is for you. You will find here a tremendously successful and popular program which we've adapted from a "quit smoking" program developed by the American Lung Association. Both the ALA's *Freedom from Smoking in 20 Days* manual and its companion booklet, *A Lifetime of Freedom from Smoking,* are maintenance guides available from your local American Lung Association affiliate.

Follow this program faithfully, and you'll be ready for chapter one in two weeks. First, however, we want you to take a few short quizzes designed to help you take a good

1

hard look at both the facts and your feelings about cigarette smoking. Tests 1 and 2 deal with the facts of life about smoking, while Test 3 will help you begin to analyze the reasons why you smoke. All the quizzes were formulated by the US Department of Health and Human Services.

When taking each test, circle the number that most accurately indicates how you feel about the statement. For example, in Test 1, if you strongly agree with the statement, then circle number four. If you strongly disagree, circle number one, etc. After completing the test, total your score as indicated and read the explanatory notes to find out what the results mean.

Test 1

	Strongly Agree	Mildly Agree	Mildly Disagree	Strongly Disagree
a. Cigarette smoking might give me a serious illness.	(4)	3	2	1
b. My cigarette smoking sets a bad example for others.	4	(3)	2	1
c. I find cigarette smoking to be a messy kind of habit.	4	(3)	2	1
d. Controlling my cigarette smoking is a challenge to me.	(4)	3	2	1
e. Smoking causes shortness of breath.	(4)	3	2	1
f. If I quit smoking cigarettes, it might influence others to stop.	4	(3)	2	1

Test 1 (*Continued*)

	Strongly Agree	Mildly Agree	Mildly Disagree	Strongly Disagree
g. Cigarettes cause damage to clothing and other personal property.	(4)	3	2	1
h. Quitting smoking would show that I have willpower.	(4)	3	2	1
i. My cigarette smoking will have a harmful effect on my health.	(4)	3	2	1
j. My cigarette smoking influences others close to me to take up or continue smoking.	4	3	(2)	1
k. If I quit smoking, my sense of taste or smell would improve.	(4)	3	2	1
l. I do not like the idea of feeling dependent on smoking.	(4)	3	2	1

How to Score

Write the number you have circled after each statement in Test 1 in the corresponding space below. Then add the scores down each column to get your totals. For example, the sum of your scores on *a, e,* and *i* gives you your score for the first column.

	Health	Examples	Esthetics	Mastery
	a _____	b __3___	c _____	d _____
	e _____	f _____	g _____	h _____
	i _____	j _____	k _____	l _____
COLUMN TOTALS:	1 _43___	2 _____	3 _____	4 _____

What Your Score Means

Test 1 was designed to measure the importance to you of each of four basic reasons for quitting. The higher you score in any one category—say health—the more important that reason is to you. A score of nine or above in one of these categories indicates that this is one of the most important reasons why you want to quit.

1. HEALTH— Research during the past twenty-five years has shown that cigarette smoking is harmful to health. Knowing this, many people have stopped smoking and many others are considering it. If your score on the health factor is nine or above, the health hazards of smoking are enough to make you want to quit now.

If your score on this factor is low (six or less), look at your scores on Test 2. They tell how much you know about the health hazard. You may be lacking important information or may even have incorrect information. If so, health considerations are not playing the important role they should be in your decision to quit.

2. EXAMPLE— Some people stop smoking because they want to set a good example to others. Parents quit to make it easier for their children to resist starting to smoke; doctors, to influence their patients; sports stars, to set an example for their

Test 2

	Strongly Agree	Mildly Agree	Mildly Disagree	Strongly Disagree
a. Cigarette smoking is not nearly as dangerous as many other health hazards.	1	(2)	3	4
b. I don't smoke enough to get any of the diseases that cigarette smoking is supposed to cause.	1	2	3	(4)
c. If a person has already smoked for many years, it probably won't do him much good to stop.	1	2	3	(4)
d. It would be hard for me to give up smoking cigarettes.	(1)	2	3	4
e. Cigarette smoking is enough of a hazard to health for something to be done about it.	1	(2)	3	4
f. The kind of cigarette I smoke is much less likely than other kinds to give me any of the diseases that smoking is supposed to cause.	1	2	3	(4)
g. As soon as a person quits smoking cigarettes he begins to recover from much of the damage that smoking has caused.	1	2	(3)	4

5

Test 2 (*Continued*)

	Strongly Agree	Mildly Agree	Mildly Disagree	Strongly Disagree
h. It would be hard for me to cut down to half the number of cigarettes I now smoke.	①	2	3	4
i. The whole problem of cigarette smoking and health is a very minor one.	1	2	3	④
j. I haven't smoked long enough to worry about the diseases that cigarette smoking is supposed to cause.	1	2	3	④
k. Quitting smoking helps a person to live longer.	①	2	3	4
l. It would be difficult for me to make any substantial change in my smoking habits.	①	2	3	4

young fans; husbands, to influence their wives and vice versa.

Such examples are an important influence on our behavior. Research shows that almost twice as many high school students smoke if both parents are smokers compared to those whose parents are nonsmokers or former smokers.

If your score is low (six or less), it may mean that you are not interested in giving up smoking in order to set an example for others. Perhaps you do not appreciate how important your example could be.

3. AESTHETICS—People who score high—nine or above—in this category recognize and are disturbed by some of the unpleasant aspects of smoking. The smell of stale smoke on their clothing, bad breath, and stains on their fingers and teeth are reason enough for them to consider breaking the habit.

4. MASTERY—If you score nine or above on this factor, you are bothered by the knowledge that you cannot control your desire to smoke. You are not your own master. Awareness of this challenge to your self-control makes you want to quit.

How to Score

Write the number you have circled after each statement in Test 2 in the corresponding space below. Then add the scores down each column to get your totals. For example, the sum of your scores on *a, e,* and *i* gives you your score for the first column.

	Importance	Personal Relevance	Value of Stopping	Ability to Stop
	a _____	b _____	c _____	d _____
	e _____	f _____	g _____	h _____
	i _____	j _____	k _____	l _____
COLUMN TOTALS:	1 _____	2 _____	3 _____	4 _____

What Your Score Means

You have just taken a test on what you believe the effects of smoking are. Your scores here give a profile of your attitudes toward the *importance* of the entire matter (column 1) and its *personal relevance* to you (column 2), as well as toward

7

the *value of stopping* (column 3) and your own *ability to stop* (column 4). If you score nine or above on any factor, that factor is influential in your desire to stop smoking. If your score is six or below, that factor will not help you—but note that you may have scored low because you lack correct information. For every factor for which you *do* have a low score, read the following explanatory material with special care.

1. IMPORTANCE—Cancer, heart disease, and respiratory diseases are all causally related to smoking, and are among the most serious to which man is exposed. You should not shrug off the evidence that they cause death and severe disability. Yet you may be doing this if your score is six or lower on this first part of Test 2.

Research has shown that about one death in every three among men who die between the ages of thirty-five and sixty is an "extra" death, because cigarette smokers have higher death rates than nonsmokers. One day of every five lost from work because of illness, one day of every seven spent in bed because of illness, one day of every eight days of restricted activity—all are "extra" because cigarette smokers suffer more disability than nonsmokers.

2. PERSONAL RELEVANCE—Some smokers kid themselves into thinking: "It can't happen to me, only the other guy." If you score six or below, you may be one of these people.

Your reasoning may go something like this: "I don't really smoke enough to be hurt by it. It takes two packs a day over a period of many years before harmful effects show up."

Unfortunately, this is not true. Even people who smoke less than half a pack a day show significantly higher death rates than comparable nonsmokers.

3. VALUE OF STOPPING—Evidence shows that there are benefits to health when you give up smoking—even if you have

8

smoked for many years. A score of six or lower indicates that you do not realize this.

There are real advantages in giving up smoking even for long-term smokers; people who quit before developing any symptoms of illness or impairment suffer lower death rates than those who continue to smoke, and they reduce their likelihood of serious illness.

People who have had heart attacks and those with stomach ulcers and chronic respiratory diseases in particular should give up smoking.

4. ABILITY TO STOP—If your score is six or lower on this part of the test, you believe that it will be hard for you to quit. But you may find encouragement in the fact that 45 million adults are now ex-smokers. You too can become one of them with some willpower and determination.

How to Score

Write the number you have circled after each statement in Test 3 in the corresponding space below. Then add the scores down each column to get your totals. For example, the sum of your scores for *a, g,* and *m* gives you your score for the first column.

	Stimu-lation	Handling	Pleasure	"Crutch"	Craving	Habit
	a ____	*b* ____	*c* ____	*d* ____	*e* ____	*f* ____
	g ____	*h* ____	*i* ____	*j* ____	*k* ____	*l* ____
	m ____	*n* ____	*o* ____	*p* ____	*q* ____	*r* ____
COLUMN TOTALS:	1 ____	2 ____	3 ____	4 ____	5 ____	6 ____

Test 3

	Frequently	Occasionally	Always	Seldom	Never
a. I smoke cigarettes to keep myself from slowing down.	5	4	3	2	(1)
b. Handling a cigarette is part of the enjoyment of smoking it.	5	4	3	(2)	1
c. Smoking cigarettes is pleasant and relaxing.	(5)	4	3	2	1
d. I light up a cigarette when I feel angry about something.	5	4	3	(2)	1
e. When I have run out of cigarettes I find it almost unbearable until I get some.	(5)	4	3	2	1
f. I smoke cigarettes automatically without even being aware of it.	5	(4)	3	2	1
g. I smoke cigarettes to stimulate me, to perk myself up.	5	(4)	3	2	1
h. Part of the enjoyment of smoking a cigarette comes from the steps I take to light up.	(5)	4	3	(2)	1
i. I find cigarettes pleasurable.	(5)	4	3	2	1

10

Statement					
j. When I feel uncomfortable or upset about something, I light up a cigarette.	5	4	3	(2)	1
k. I am very much aware of the fact when I am not smoking a cigarette.	5	4	3	(2)	1
l. I light up a cigarette without realizing I still have one burning in the ashtray.	5	4	3	(2)	1
m. I smoke cigarettes to give me a "lift."	5	4	3	(2)	1
n. When I smoke a cigarette, part of the enjoyment is watching the smoke as I exhale it.	(5)	4	(3)	2	1
o. I want a cigarette most when I am comfortable and relaxed.	5	4	3	2	1
p. When I feel "blue" or want to take my mind off cares and worries, I smoke cigarettes.	5	4	3	(2)	1
q. I get a real gnawing hunger for a cigarette when I haven't smoked for a while.	(5)	4	3	2	1
r. I've found a cigarette in my mouth and didn't remember putting it there.	5	4	3	(2)	1

What Your Score Means

In this test examining reasons why you smoke, a score of eleven or above on any factor indicates that it is an important source of satisfaction for you. The higher you score (fifteen is the highest), the more important a particular factor is in your smoking and the more useful the discussion of that factor can be in your attempt to quit. If you do not score high on any of the six factors, chances are that you do not smoke very much or have not been smoking for many years. If so, giving up smoking—and staying off—should be easy for you.

1. STIMULATION—If you score high or fairly high on this factor, it means that you are one of those smokers who is stimulated by the cigarette—you feel that it helps wake you up, organize your energies, and keep you going.

2. HANDLING—If you score high in this test, you smoke partly out of a nervous habit. Handling things can be satisfying, but there are many ways to keep your hands busy without lighting up or playing with a cigarette.

3. PLEASURE—It is not always easy to find out whether you use that cigarette to feel good—that is, if you get real, honest pleasure out of smoking (column 3)—or to keep from feeling so bad (column 4). About two-thirds of smokers score high or fairly high in the "accentuation of pleasure" category, and about half of those also score as high or higher in the "crutch" column.

4. "CRUTCH," OR REDUCTION OF NEGATIVE FEELINGS— Many smokers use the cigarette as a kind of crutch in moments of stress or discomfort. But the heavy smoker, the person who tries to handle severe personal problems by smoking many

times a day, is apt to discover that cigarettes do not help in dealing with problems effectively.

5. CRAVING—Quitting smoking is difficult for the person who scores high on this factor, since it indicates the possibility of a physical dependence. For the addicted smoker, the craving for the next cigarette begins to build up the moment the last cigarette is put out.

6. HABIT—If you are smoking out of habit, you no longer get much satisfaction from your cigarettes. You just light them frequently without even realizing you are doing so.

Why Do You Smoke?

Okay, you've now completed the tests. Whether you realize it or not, you've already taken the first step in our two-week stop-smoking program.

One of the keys to giving up cigarettes is to learn why or what "triggers," or sets off, your urge to smoke. The important thing to remember is that no two smokers are alike in the reasons why they smoke. That's why the first five days of this two-week program are preparation days. During this time you will learn more than you may even want to know about your individual smoking habits. Armed with that knowledge, you can begin to kick the habit.

Test 3 gave you a general idea about why you, as an individual, smoke—whether from dependence, habit, desire for stimulation, etc. We want you to get more specific now and determine what particular activities, places, or people trigger your desire to light up.

During the first five days of this program we want you to wrap your pack of cigarettes with paper and rubber bands.

DAILY TALLY SHEET

	Time	Place or Activity	With Whom	Need (1–5)	Mood or Reason
1.					
2.					
3.					
4.					
5.					
6.					
7.					
8.					

9. _____

10. _____

11. _____

12. _____

13. _____

14. _____

15. _____

16. _____

17. _____

18. _____

19. _____

20. _____

Each time you light up, note the time of day, what you are doing at that moment, whom you are with, how you are feeling, and how important that cigarette is to you on a scale of one to five. A five indicates an intense desire. A one is a low-level need. Each night transfer these results to the tally sheets we have provided you with. This is *important* preparation, so follow the rules faithfully with each and every cigarette you smoke.

Furthermore, we also want you to list all the reasons you want to quit smoking. Some of the most common reasons are discussed in Test 1, so you might want to go back and review your answers. Now please don't get the idea that we want you to include only the major reasons like health. Be sure to list some really personal irritations with smoking like having to rush out in the middle of the night to some gas station when you discover that you are out of smokes. Or note with disgust the time you burned a hole in Aunt Sara's party dress when you were dancing with her at your daughter's wedding. Or remember how embarrassing it was to get caught by your nonsmoking boss in a no-smoking area because you just couldn't wait any longer to light up. Now, every night before going to bed, repeat one of these reasons ten times.

Chances are smoking is pretty automatic to you by now. Sometimes you may light up without even realizing it! That's why during these preparation days we want you to really be aware of each and every cigarette you smoke. From now on, we also want you to hold each cigarette you smoke in the hand you don't usually use. We also would like you to put your packs of cigarettes in an unfamiliar place—like the garage or porch.

If you're at work, you might try leaving them in the glove compartment of your car. Make them hard to get at. You might even think about putting those cigarettes in a jar equipped with a child's safety cap. If all this doesn't help and you continue to light up many times during the day without thinking about it, try to look in the mirror each time you put a match to your cigarette.

From now on, you're only to buy one pack of cigarettes at a time—that means no more cartons! Also, no stockpiling of cigarettes is allowed. You've got to wait until one pack is empty before purchasing another.

Now is also the time to begin conditioning yourself physically. It is crucial that you start an exercise program. It will become even more important when you're withdrawing from the effects of nicotine. We'll be talking a lot about that later in this book. To get you started on an exercise program, however, you may want to read through Chapter 5, "These Boots Are Made for Walking."

During this preparation period, it is also important that you begin to modify your eating patterns. Make a small change now. For example, drink milk, which is frequently considered incompatible with smoking. We also want you to begin to learn how to relax at this point. You might want to start practicing the deep-breathing exercises described in Chapter 7, "How Do You Spell Relief?"

Let someone you care about know that you've decided to quit smoking. The American Lung Association suggests writing a short statement including some of the reasons why you're going to stop. Now put that statement in an envelope and mail it to a friend or relative. Doing this should strengthen your sense of commitment.

Another important step for you to follow during this preparation period is to begin to select rewards for not smoking. Chances are cigarettes have been a big part in your past reward system. You probably rewarded yourself with a cigarette on a housework break, after a difficult business deal, or at the five-o'clock whistle for making it through another work day.

But what we want you to do now is to think up some

rewards you can use while going through this "quit smoking" program. Have fun, be imaginative and even silly—after all, that's what these rewards are all about. A few such rewards for sticking with the program may be on the expensive side, but there's no need to go overboard. A vacation would be in order for completing the entire program, but not for eliminating one cigarette from your daily quota.

Above all, remember that rewards don't all have to be material. It really is true that some of the best things in life are free. How about treating yourself to a lazy weekend morning by sleeping late, reading, or watching television. But remember, to enjoy such a morning you really have to earn it. In other words, no cheating! Reward yourself—treat yourself to a great time—if and only if you achieve a goal toward becoming a nonsmoker.

When you begin the action plan, each and every day that you complete the program or activity for that day, reward yourself. You may find yourself trying to think up a lot of rewards in the next nine days, so here are a few ideas to help you out.

- Use only new golf balls when you play. The same goes for the balls you use in tennis.
- Purchase that new tennis racket or golf club you've always wanted.
- Call a friend you've been meaning to call and have lunch or dinner.
- Get your hair done.
- Enjoy a massage.
- Eat dinner at your favorite restaurant.
- Take a long, leisurely walk.
- Visit a favorite museum or take a drive out to the country.

A good idea suggested by the American Lung Association is to choose a buddy to go through the next week of the program with you. A buddy is that special someone who will act as your cheerleader for at least the next seven days. You and your pal should be in contact at least once a day either in person or by telephone.

It's important that your friend be someone who really roots for your efforts. You certainly don't need any nagging or a doubting Thomas at this stage. The ALA further recommends that your buddy be someone who has never smoked, or someone who hasn't smoked in at least a year.

Now, before we get to day one of the program, we want you to thoroughly review the tally sheets you've been faithfully filling out for the past five days. Go back and underline the listings that appear *most often* on your tally sheets. This will help you determine your day-in and day-out smoking pattern. Now take a look at the pattern-breaking sheet we have also provided you with. Transfer your tally-sheet situations over to the pattern-breaking sheet under the column entitled, "Trigger situation." If any of the situations for smoking were avoidable, put an *A* next to them in the appropriate column. If they were not, put an *NA* in the same column.

For example, on your tally sheet you've listed your first cigarette of the day as taking place at the kitchen table while you were relaxing with your family over a cup of coffee. Since it's the first cigarette of the day, you rated it as an intense need and scored it as a number five. Now transfer that situation to your pattern-breaking sheet. You've decided that situation was not avoidable, so you jot down *NA* in the appropriate column. You must now devise a coping technique so that this pattern is not repeated day after day.

We say "you," because, as we've already learned, every smoker is an individual and smokes for a different reason. Coping techniques operate that way also. What may work

PATTERN-BREAKING SHEET

Trigger Situation: Place or Activity; with Whom; Mood or Reason	Need	A or NA	Method of Avoiding Situation	Coping Techniques
1.				
2.				
3.				
4.				
5.				
6.				
7.				

8.

9.

10.

11.

12.

13.

14.

15.

16.

17.

18.

19.

20.

for someone else will not necessarily work for you. Some coping techniques you may choose include doing stretching exercises or other physical activity. You might want to chew some sugarless gum or read a book. In short, do anything that you normally would not associate with smoking. Jot down the coping technique you have selected in the last column on the pattern-breaking sheet. Also, if possible, list a method or methods for avoiding that kitchen-table scenario—and its accompanying temptation to smoke—in the first place.

Let's take another example. You've listed on your tally sheet that you took a friend to dinner. The service was slow and you fell into an impatient mood. To pass the time, you smoked a cigarette. However, the need was not extremely intense, so you rated it as a two.

Transferring this information to the pattern-breaking sheet, you noted the situation as avoidable (*A*). Why? Because in thinking about that dinner you realize that your impatience stemmed from selecting a restaurant far from home. The hour was getting late and you began to worry about having to travel a long distance by yourself. You could easily have avoided such a smoking-pressure situation by having a pleasant dinner with your friend nearer to home. Make note of that in the column on methods of avoiding such smoking-trigger situations.

From now on you must make a conscious effort to avoid these types of situations. This may be the perfect time, for example, to visit those museums or that library you've neglected for the last few years. It is a rare museum, after all, which allows smoking, and that's the whole point of choosing such an activity. Also, if you find yourself in a restaurant, it would be a good idea to sit in the no-smoking section if there is one. Movies, plays, and concerts are also good activities because smoking is discouraged where they take place.

At this point let's take a final look at each of your regular day-in, day-out cigarette patterns. Transfer them all to your pattern-breaking sheet. Determine whether each situation in which you lit up was either avoidable or not avoidable. Devise either a coping technique or a method of avoiding such a situation in the future. Make notes in the appropriate columns.

Now let's get ready to begin the real nitty-gritty aspect of this program. But first, a reminder. We want you, *each and every day of this program,* to begin a new tally sheet and transfer its information to your pattern-breaking chart at day's end. And remember to repeat ten times each reason you have for not wanting to smoke. Get involved in some regular physical activity, practice breathing exercises to help you relax, and make access to your cigarettes more difficult. Remember, also, to smoke using an unaccustomed hand. (Another excellent technique for helping to rid yourself of the desire to light up after a meal is to brush your teeth immediately after eating. That toothpaste flavor often does the trick.

Okay, let's get ready for day six . . .

Day Six

ONE— The first thing you're going to do today is change brands of cigarettes. Look at the Federal Trade Commission chart we've provided you with at the end of the introduction and choose a brand that's lower in tar and nicotine than the cigarettes you are presently smoking. During the next week you're going to gradually ease off on tar and nicotine levels in preparation for the big day when you put out your last cigarette.

TWO— Refer to your pattern-breaking sheet and select a trigger that you've rated as a one or two. Choose a coping technique that you'll use. Now eliminate that cigarette from those you'll smoke today.

THREE— From today on, cut back on the amount of coffee you drink. We all know that coffee goes with cigarettes, so easing up on the java for a while should make it easier to ease up on the cigarettes too.

FOUR— Make it a point to spend time with nonsmokers. One of the most powerful triggers is other smokers lighting up. Of course, we're not asking you to sever relationships, just minimize the time you spend with your smoking friends for a while.

If you have successfully completed the action plan for this day, reward yourself!

Day Seven

ONE— Refer, again, to the Federal Trade Commission chart and choose a brand that's lower in tar and nicotine than yesterday's brand. Use that brand.

TWO— Return to your pattern-breaking sheet and select two triggers that make you want to smoke when you're alone, and which you've rated a one or a two. Eliminate those cigarettes today!

THREE— From now on we want you to smoke less of your cigarettes. Today, smoke each cigarette to the halfway point and put it out. Draw a line at the halfway point so that you won't smoke past it.

FOUR— One more thing for today—and this is the easy part. Figure out how much you're going to save each year by not letting your money go up in smoke. To do that, multiply by 365 what you spend on cigarettes in a day. It's probably a lot more than you think. That chunk of change could buy you something pretty special. Consider what you might like to buy with that extra money.

If you have successfully completed all the action-plan activities for day seven, reward yourself. You deserve it!

Day Eight

ONE— Once again, change brands to a cigarette that's lower in tar and nicotine than yesterday's brand.

TWO— We're going to step things up a bit today and eliminate three cigarettes from your smoking pattern. As you did yesterday, choose triggers that make you want to smoke when you're alone. But this time select triggers that you rate as a two or three.

THREE— Today we also want you to start a butt jar. Get a large jar with a tight lid. Put all—and we mean all—your cigarette butts in that jar. This means that you must save those butts from work, restaurants, and, we're sorry to say, even those you've squashed out on the sidewalk. Be sure and put that jar right by your bed so you can gaze upon it first thing in the morning and at night.

How did you do on day eight? Did you complete all your activities? If so, remember to reward yourself.

Day Nine

ONE— We're really going to test you today. Why? Because we think you're ready. We want you to eliminate another cigarette from your smoking pattern, but choose a trigger that causes an intense craving—say a four or a five.

TWO— Now we know that for us smokers, inhaling a cigarette is a pretty automatic thing. But from now on we really want you to be aware of it. Try to think about how hard you're pulling on that cigarette, and from now on try to do less and less pulling each time you inhale.

THREE— From today on we want you to delay lighting up your cigarette for at least a minute or two. During this time try to change your activity or talk to someone. You may find that you can do without that cigarette.

FOUR— Sorry, but from now on you don't carry any matches or cigarette lighters. If you have to bum lights every time you want a smoke, we know that's pretty inconvenient and that's just the way we want it.

How did day nine go? Reward yourself if you successfully completed all your activities.

Day Ten

ONE—_ We're willing to bet that you did so well yesterday in eliminating that intense-craving cigarette from your pattern, that today you're ready for an even greater challenge. So, let's up the ante a bit. Today we want you to eliminate *two* intense-craving cigarettes from your pattern. Choose one trigger that operates when you're alone and one with other people.

TWO— Today is the day that you get rid of all your smoking accessories. We mean even that beautiful cigarette case that you got from a friend last Christmas.

THREE—This is also the day that you begin turning down any cigarettes people may offer you. When you're out of cigarettes you're out of cigarettes. You'll just have to wait until day eleven to smoke.

Did you successfully meet the challenges of day ten? Then it's reward time.

Day Eleven

ONE—Switch brands once again to an even lower-tar-and-nicotine cigarette than you smoked yesterday.

TWO—By now you're an old pro at eliminating intense-craving cigarettes from your smoking pattern. Today we're going to be easy on you and just ask that you eliminate two more intense triggers. Once again, choose one that operates when you're alone and one with other people.

THREE—Today speak up and be counted among the almost smokeless. Tell everyone and anyone who will listen that you're quitting smoking—friends, co-workers, relatives, and even the elevator operator. Discuss your top five reasons for quitting and target date—it's only two days away, you know!

FOUR—We hope that for the last couple of days you've delayed lighting up your cigarettes for a few minutes. Now we want you to delay lighting up for a full five minutes. If you must, keep track of the time with a watch.

Are the days getting any easier for you? We hope so. For successfully completing today's activities, don't neglect that award.

Day Twelve

ONE— We want you to change brands again. The good news? Today is the last day you'll be switching brands. You're almost there!

TWO— Eliminate two more cigarettes from your pattern— intense-need ones, of course. Go after the intense urges that you feel when you're alone. The good news today is that this is the last day you'll be referring to your pattern-breaking sheet.

THREE— Figure out the number of cigarettes you'll be smoking today and take only 80 percent of that number with you. When you're out of smokes you're out of smokes, and you can't have any more cigarettes for this day.

Really reward yourself today if you're still on track with this program—you're almost home!

Day Thirteen

ONE— Today when you smoke we don't want you to do anything but smoke. Don't read, watch television, drink coffee, or talk to anyone. Pretty boring, isn't it?

TWO— Cut your number of cigarettes today by 20 percent. At the end of the day get rid of all your remaining cigarettes. As you put out that last cigarette of the day, tell yourself: "I've just put out the last cigarette of my life. I'm now a nonsmoker."

Of course the word for today is *reward! reward! reward!*

Day Fourteen

The big day has finally arrived! The first thing to do is to flush the nicotine out of your system fast, and that means drink a lot of water, fruit juices, etc. It is also a great day to visit the dentist and have your teeth cleaned. Get rid of those tobacco-stained teeth once and for all.

As a matter of fact, pay special attention to your entire appearance today. You're a winner and you deserve to look like one!

But don't worry, we're not going to leave you here. This is only day one of your whole new life. Let's face it, you've still got some mountains to climb, but that's what this book is all about—surviving and winning the battle against nicotine addiction. And we'll be with you all the way.

From now on we're going to be talking survival as a new ex-smoker, so read on, MacDuff . . .

Tar, Nicotine, and Carbon Monoxide Content of Various Brands of Domestic Cigarettes Tested by FTC Method

(Increasing Order of Nicotine)

Brand Name	Type	Tar*	Nicotine†	Carbon Monoxide‡
Cambridge	king size; filter; hard pack	§	§	§
Carlton	king size; filter; hard pack	§	§	§
Now	king size; filter; hard pack	§	§	§
Now 100	100mm; filter; hard pack	§	§	§
Carlton 100	100mm; filter; menthol; hard pack	1	0.1	§
Carlton 100	100mm; filter; hard pack	1	0.1	§
Cambridge	king size; filter	1	0.1	1
Carlton	king size; filter; menthol	1	0.1	1
Now	king size; filter	1	0.1	1
Now	king size; filter; menthol	1	0.1	1
Benson & Hedges	reg. size; filter; hard pack	1	0.1	2
Carlton	king size; filter	1	0.1	2
Kool Ultra	king size; filter; menthol	2	0.2	1
Now 100	100mm; filter; menthol	2	0.2	1
Now 100	100mm; filter	2	0.2	2

* "Tar"—milligrams total particulate matter less nicotine and water per cigarette.
† Nicotine total alkaloids reported in milligrams per cigarette.
‡ Carbon monoxide reported in milligrams per cigarette.
§—Indicates "tar" below 0.5 mg.; nicotine below 0.05 mg.; or carbon monoxide below 0.5 mg. per cigarette.
Source: US Department of Health and Human Services.

Brand	Type			
Kent III	king size; filter	3	0.3	3
Triumph	king size; filter; menthol	3	0.3	3
Iceberg 100	100mm; filter; menthol	3	0.3	4
Lucky 100	100mm; filter	3	0.3	4
Merit Ultra Lights	king size; filter	4	0.3	4
Merit Ultra Lights	king size; filter; menthol	4	0.3	4
Merit Ultra Lights 100	100mm; filter; menthol	4	0.3	4
Triumph	king size; filter	3	0.4	3
Salem Ultra	king size; filter; menthol	4	0.4	4
Kent III 100	100mm; filter	4	0.4	5
Triumph 100	100mm; filter	4	0.4	5
Doral II	king size; filter	5	0.4	3
Doral II	100mm; filter; menthol	5	0.4	3
Kool Ultra 100	100mm; filter; menthol	5	0.4	4
Tareyton Lights	king size; filter	5	0.4	4
Cambridge 100	100mm; filter	5	0.4	5
Carlton 100	100mm; filter; menthol	5	0.4	5
Carlton 100	100mm; filter	5	0.4	5
Salem Ultra 100	100mm; filter; menthol	5	0.4	5
True	king size; filter	5	0.4	5
True	king size; filter; menthol	5	0.4	5
Vantage Ultra Lights	king size; filter	5	0.4	6
Vantage Ultra Lights	king size; filter; menthol	5	0.4	6
Vantage Ultra Lights 100	100mm; filter	5	0.4	6
Winston Ultra	king size; filter	5	0.4	6
Winston Ultra 100	100mm; filter	5	0.4	6
Vantage Ultra Lights 100	100mm; filter; menthol	5	0.4	7

Tar, Nicotine, and Carbon Monoxide Content of Various Brands of Domestic Cigarettes Tested by FTC Method (*Continued*)

Brand Name	Type	Tar*	Nicotine†	Carbon Monoxide‡
Triumph 100	100mm; filter; menthol	4	0.5	5
Carlton 120	120mm; filter; menthol	6	0.5	4
Decade	king size; filter	6	0.5	5
Decade	king size; filter; menthol	6	0.5	5
Benson & Hedges Ultra Light	100mm; filter; menthol; hard pack	6	0.5	6
Benson & Hedges Ultra Light	100mm; filter; hard pack	6	0.5	6
Merit Ultra Lights 100	100mm; filter	6	0.5	7
Bright	king size; filter; menthol	6	0.5	8
Carlton 120	120mm; filter	6	0.6	5
Omni 100	100mm; filter; menthol	7	0.6	6
Pall Mall Extra Light	king size; filter	7	0.6	6
Tareyton Long Lights 100	100mm; filter	7	0.6	7
More Lights 100	100mm; filter; menthol; hard pack	7	0.6	8
Salem Slim Lights 100	100mm; filter; menthol; hard pack	7	0.6	8
Bright 100	100mm; filter; menthol	7	0.6	10
Virginia Slims Lights 100	100mm; filter; menthol; hard pack	8	0.6	7
Camel Lights	king size; filter; hard pack	8	0.6	8
More Lights 100	100mm; filter; hard pack	8	0.6	8
True 100	100mm; filter	8	0.6	8
Virginia Slims Lights 100	100mm; filter; hard pack	8	0.6	8

Brand	Description			
Salem Lights	king size; filter; menthol	8	0.6	9
True 100	100mm; filter; menthol	8	0.6	9
Camel Lights	king size; filter	8	0.6	10
Parliament Lights	king size; filter; hard pack	9	0.6	9
Winston Lights	king size; filter	9	0.6	10
Merit	king size; filter	9	0.6	11
Merit	king size; filter; menthol	9	0.6	11
Belair	king size; filter; menthol	9	0.7	9
Golden Lights	king size; filter	9	0.7	9
Golden Lights	king size; filter; menthol	9	0.7	9
Golden Lights 100	100mm; filter; menthol	9	0.7	9
Newport Lights	king size; filter; menthol	9	0.7	9
Newport Lights	king size; filter; menthol; hard pack	9	0.7	9
Raleigh Lights	king size; filter	9	0.7	9
Belair 100	100mm; filter; menthol	9	0.7	10
Kool Lights	king size; filter; menthol	9	0.7	10
Viceroy Rich Lights	king size; filter	9	0.7	10
Salem Lights 100	100mm; filter; menthol	9	0.7	11
Vantage	king size; filter	9	0.7	12
Vantage 100	100mm; filter	9	0.7	12
Parliament Lights	king size; filter	10	0.7	9
Benson & Hedges Lights 100	100mm; filter; menthol	10	0.7	11
Marlboro Lights	king size; filter; hard pack	10	0.7	11
Northwind	king size; filter; menthol	10	0.7	11
Benson & Hedges Lights 100	100mm; filter	10	0.7	12
Merit 100	100mm; filter; menthol	10	0.7	12
Vantage	king size; filter; menthol	10	0.7	13

Tar, Nicotine, and Carbon Monoxide Content of Various Brands of Domestic Cigarettes Tested by FTC Method (*Continued*)

Brand Name	Type	Tar*	Nicotine†	Carbon Monoxide‡
Marlboro Lights	king size; filter	11	0.7	11
Northwind 100	100mm; filter; menthol	11	0.7	11
Marlboro Lights 100	100mm; filter	11	0.7	12
Merit 100	100mm; filter	11	0.7	13
L & M Lights 100	100mm; filter	8	0.8	5
L & M Lights 100	100mm; filter; menthol	8	0.8	6
L & M Lights	king size; filter	9	0.8	7
Pall Mall Light 100	100mm; filter	9	0.8	7
Golden Lights 100	100mm; filter	9	0.8	9
Kool Lights 100	100mm; filter; menthol	10	0.8	9
Newport Lights 100	100mm; filter; menthol	10	0.8	10
Satin 100	100mm; filter	10	0.8	10
Old Gold Lights	king size; filter	10	0.8	11
Satin 100	100mm; filter; menthol	10	0.8	11
Raleigh Lights 100	100mm; filter	10	0.8	12
Viceroy Rich Lights 100	100mm; filter	10	0.8	12
Lucky Strike	king size; filter	11	0.8	11
Kool Milds	king size; filter; menthol	11	0.8	12
Lucky Strike	king size; filter; hard pack	11	0.8	12
Kool Milds 100	100mm; filter; menthol	11	0.8	13

Brand	Description			
Multifilter	king size; filter	12	0.8	11
Camel Lights 100	100mm; filter	12	0.8	14
Winston Lights 100	100mm; filter	12	0.8	14
Multifilter	king size; filter; menthol	13	0.8	11
Alpine	king size; filter; menthol	14	0.8	14
Parliament Lights 100	100mm; filter	11	0.9	10
Rebel	king size; filter	11	0.9	12
Kent	king size; filter	12	0.9	11
Kent	king size; filter; hard pack	12	0.9	12
Lark Lights	king size; filter	13	0.9	12
L & M	king size; filter	14	0.9	13
L & M	king size; filter; hard pack	14	0.9	13
Saratoga 120	120mm; filter; hard pack	14	0.9	14
Marlboro	king size; filter; menthol; hard pack	15	0.9	13
Marlboro	king size; filter; menthol	15	0.9	14
Galaxy	king size; filter	15	0.9	15
Viceroy	king size; filter	15	0.9	17
Silva Thins 100	100mm; filter	12	1.0	9
Silva Thins 100	100mm; filter; menthol	12	1.0	9
Rebel 100	100mm; filter	12	1.0	13
Pall Mall Light 100	100mm; filter; menthol	13	1.0	12
Eve Lights 100	100mm; filter	13	1.0	13
Eve Lights 100	100mm; filter; menthol	13	1.0	13
Newport Red	king size; filter	13	1.0	15
Newport Red	king size; filter; hard pack	13	1.0	15
Eve Lights 120	120mm; filter; menthol; hard pack	14	1.0	11
Kent 100	100mm; filter	14	1.0	12

Tar, Nicotine, and Carbon Monoxide Content of Various Brands of Domestic Cigarettes Tested by FTC Method (*Continued*)

Brand Name	Type	Tar*	Nicotine†	Carbon Monoxide‡
Lark	king size; filter	14	1.0	13
Lark Lights 100	100mm; filter	14	1.0	14
Saratoga 120	120mm; filter; menthol; hard pack	14	1.0	14
L & M 100	100mm; filter	14	1.0	15
Tareyton	king size; filter	14	1.0	15
Tareyton 100	100mm; filter	14	1.0	15
Viceroy Super Long 100	100mm; filter	14	1.0	16
Salem 100	100mm; filter; menthol	15	1.0	13
Camel	king size; filter	15	1.0	14
Virginia Slims 100	100mm; filter	15	1.0	14
Virginia Slims 100	100mm; filter; menthol	15	1.0	14
Chesterfield	king size; filter	15	1.0	15
Chesterfield 100	100mm; filter	15	1.0	16
Kool Super Longs 100	100mm; filter; menthol	15	1.0	16
Raleigh	king size; filter	15	1.0	16
Winston	king size; filter	15	1.0	16
Salem	king size; filter; menthol	16	1.0	14
Winston International 100	100mm; filter; hard pack	16	1.0	14
Winston	king size; filter; hard pack	16	1.0	15
Montclair	king size; filter; menthol	16	1.0	16
Marlboro	king size; filter	17	1.0	16
Picayune	reg. size; nonfilter	18	1.0	14

Brand	Description			
Spring 100	100mm; filter; menthol	19	1.0	16
Eve Lights 120	120mm; filter; hard pack	14	1.1	11
Benson & Hedges	king size; filter; hard pack	15	1.1	13
St. Moritz 100	100mm; filter	15	1.1	14
St. Moritz 100	100mm; filter; menthol	15	1.1	14
Kool	king size; filter; menthol; hard pack	16	1.1	15
Lark 100	100mm; filter	16	1.1	15
Raleigh 100	100mm; filter	16	1.1	16
Winston 100	100mm; filter	16	1.1	16
Newport	king size; filter; menthol; hard pack	16	1.1	17
Benson & Hedges 100	100mm; filter; menthol; hard pack	17	1.1	15
Benson & Hedges 100	100mm; filter; hard pack	17	1.1	15
Kool	king size; filter; menthol	17	1.1	15
Marlboro	king size; filter; hard pack	17	1.1	15
Marlboro 100	100mm; filter	17	1.1	15
Marlboro 100	100mm; filter; hard pack	17	1.1	15
Benson & Hedges 100	100mm; filter	17	1.1	16
Benson & Hedges 100	100mm; filter; menthol	17	1.1	16
Newport	king size; filter; menthol	17	1.1	17
Pall Mall	king size; filter	17	1.1	17
More 120	120mm; filter	17	1.1	20
Kent 100	100mm; filter; menthol	15	1.2	13
More 120	120mm; filter; menthol	15	1.2	18
Pall Mall 100	100mm; filter	16	1.2	15
Half & Half	king size; filter	17	1.2	16
Old Gold Filter	king size; filter	18	1.2	18
Camel	reg. size; nonfilter	20	1.2	12
Kool	reg. size; nonfilter; menthol	20	1.2	14

Tar, Nicotine, and Carbon Monoxide Content of Various Brands of Domestic Cigarettes Tested by FTC Method (*Concluded*)

Brand Name	Type	Tar*	Nicotine†	Carbon Monoxide‡
Chesterfield	reg. size; nonfilter	21	1.2	12
Tall 120	120mm; filter; menthol	17	1.3	16
Long Johns 120	120mm; filter; menthol	17	1.3	18
Long Johns 120	120mm; filter	18	1.3	19
Philip Morris	reg. size; nonfilter	22	1.3	13
Max 120	120mm; filter	18	1.4	17
Max 120	120mm; filter; menthol	18	1.4	17
Newport 100	100mm; filter; menthol	20	1.4	19
Old Gold Filter 100	100mm; filter	20	1.4	19
Lucky Strike	reg. size; nonfilter	24	1.4	16
Pall Mall	king size; nonfilter	24	1.4	16
Raleigh	king size; nonfilter	24	1.4	17
Tall 120	120mm; filter	19	1.5	19
English Ovals	reg. size; nonfilter; hard pack	22	1.5	12
Chesterfield	king size; nonfilter	25	1.5	15
Old Gold Straight	king size; nonfilter	26	1.6	18
Philip Morris Commander	king size; nonfilter	27	1.6	15
Herbert Tareyton	king size; nonfilter	26	1.7	16
Bull Durham	king size; filter	28	1.8	23
Players	reg. size; nonfilter; hard pack	27	1.9	15
English Ovals	king size; nonfilter; hard pack	29	2.1	15

O · N · E

BODY LANGUAGE: THE ABCs OF WITHDRAWAL

Now that your body realizes you're no longer going to supply it with its daily nicotine fix, it's going to put you through a lot of changes.

For example, you may begin to experience sensations such as light-headedness or even some dizziness. But keep in mind that such discomforts will be of short duration. Meanwhile, while such withdrawal symptoms run their course, focus on the positive side of things. Even while your body begins to act like a spoiled child deprived of its favorite plaything, it is at the same time beginning to heal itself from all the damage caused by smoking.

Other symptoms you may experience within the first five days after giving up cigarettes are nervousness, some irritability, and a feeling of being "high" or "in a fog." Believe it or not, this is a positive development. It means that your lungs are repairing themselves from years of smoke damage and are drawing in healthy doses of oxygen! Again, these symptoms usually don't last more than a week.

Many new ex-smokers also report feelings of exhaustion, a prickling in the fingers, some nausea, constipation, and diarrhea—although not everybody who quits smoking is affected this way.

It may all sound pretty terrible, but we need to emphasize that researchers have found that all these reactions disappear or diminish considerably within four weeks—so hang in there. In fact, even the craving for a cigarette—one of the worst demons we new ex-smokers must wrestle with—usually reaches its peak within the first twenty-four hours and diminishes over a seven-day period of time.

But a word of caution. That craving for tobacco will slowly return, and you will have to draw upon all your willpower for at least eight more weeks—perhaps longer—until you regain control of the situation. How long these cravings last, of course, is dependent on how heavy a smoker you were.

Interestingly enough, studies indicate that your sudden desire for a smoke will last in its most intense form for no more than five minutes—a perfect time to practice the breathing exercises and other techniques described later in this book and designed to help you weather such storms. You may also be interested to know that such cravings are at their strongest during the evening hours.

There are other annoying little games your body will play with you during the withdrawal process. If you are like most new ex-smokers, you will probably experience feelings of depression, irritability, stress, increased boredom, mood swings, and even downright anger. But to be forewarned is to be forearmed, and we're going to arm you with some pretty solid coping techniques for these emotions a little later on in this book. Meanwhile, we've provided you with a chart (at the end of this chapter) to keep track of these various mood changes. It is important to keep such a chart because, unless you know exactly where, when, and why you are experiencing such emotions, it can be very difficult to cope with them.

Now let's turn to the positive changes which take effect inside your body within minutes of putting out that last cigarette. Incredibly enough, within twenty minutes of not smoking your heart function, circulation, and even your motor coordination all begin to improve.

Also within twenty minutes of not smoking, blood pressure, pulse rate, and the body temperature of hands and feet return to normal levels, according to studies undertaken by the American Cancer Society. And at the same time, accumulated tar in your respiratory system actually begins to dissolve.

An interesting study done in 1967 by the Sloan-Kettering Institute for Cancer Research demonstrated that one of the most striking of the changes that take place after the cessation of smoking is the virtual disappearance of "smoker's cough." Not only that, but 51 percent of the former smokers who participated in the study also reported that they no longer found themselves continuously clearing their throats. Furthermore, researchers noted an "impressive decrease" in complaints of shortness of breath by ex-smokers who participated in the study. All these changes took place in an astounding four-week period of time!

Let's get back to the timetable of healthful improvements in your body once you quit smoking. After only eight hours of going smokeless, carbon monoxide levels in the bloodstream return to normal as does the oxygen level in your blood. In just two days of not smoking, your damaged nerve endings begin regrowing, and the ability to taste and smell are increased.

There's more! Researchers have found that after seventy-two hours without a cigarette your bronchial tubes begin to regain their elasticity—which makes breathing a whole lot eas-

EMOTIONS CHART

	Time	Place	Activity	With Whom	Mood	Urge for Cigarette/Food
1.						
2.						
3.						
4.						
5.						
6.						
7.						
8.						

9. _____

10. _____

11. _____

12. _____

13. _____

14. _____

15. _____

16. _____

17. _____

18. _____

19. _____

20. _____

ier—while your lung capacity increases. In fact, the functioning of the lungs improves an amazing 30 percent within only two to three months of not smoking.

The news keeps getting better the longer you don't smoke. After one to nine months of remaining smoke-free, not only has your circulation vastly improved but so have any problems you may have had with shortness of breath and sinus congestion. Also during this time the damaged cilia in your lungs are regrowing, which means you will have less chance of an infection in that organ. Sound great? It is!

Even better news is that after five years without cigarettes (yes, you'll get there), the lung cancer death rate for the average one-pack-per-day smoker decreases from 137 per 100,000 people to 72 per 100,000 people. After ten years, that rate drops to approximately 12 deaths per 100,000 people—which is about how many people die from lung cancer who have never smoked.

We are now gazing even further into your future as a nonsmoker. Ten years after you quit, precancerous cells will have been replaced, and the possibility of cancer of the mouth, larynx, esophagus, bladder, kidney, and pancreas will have all been significantly decreased.

Needless to say, this process is a continuing one. But it may take a bit more convincing to keep you on this healthy path. So now let's take a closer look at the health hazards of smoking, should you decide to stray off the path . . .

T · W · O

SMOKE GETS IN
YOUR EYES

*"Warning: The Surgeon General Has Determined That Cigarette
Smoking Is Hazardous to Your Health."*

Uncle Sam wasn't kidding when, back in 1970, he forced the
giant tobacco companies to carry this warning on every package
of cigarettes. The government wasn't kidding then about the
hazards of smoking, nor is it less serious today about that
subject—to the extent of even banning cigarette commercials
from television. Cigarettes have been, and continue to be, public
health enemy number one in America.

Consider yourself lucky that you were finally able to read
the writing on the wall—you and the 45 million other former
smokers who in the past twenty-one years have quit the habit.
Now if only the other 54 million people in this country who
do smoke would do the same! In deciding to stop risking your
life, you will reap many positive benefits, including a harvest
of good health.

The value of being an ex-smoker is enormous when you stop to consider how many thousands of people needlessly die each year from smoking-related diseases. The irony, of course, is that smoking is the largest *preventable* cause of death in this country today. Nonetheless, warnings go unheeded. It is as if smokers have convinced themselves that such statistics only apply to other people—not themselves.

If you are still a smoker while reading this book, the following statistics may help convince you to quit the habit once and for all.

- Each year some 80,000 deaths from lung cancer are directly attributed to smoking.

- Smoking is also responsible for 22,000 other cancer-related deaths in this country each year.

- As many as 225,000 deaths in the United States are reported each year from cardiovascular disease linked to cigarette smoking.

- Each year in this country approximately 19,000 people die from chronic pulmonary disease—every single case related to smoking.

If you are an ex-smoker and have just read these statistics, a sigh of relief is in order. Do you see what you've rescued yourself from? But we're not through yet . . .

Cigarette smoking is, as the above statistics clearly indicate, the *major single cause* of cancer mortality in the United States today. Tobacco's contribution to all cancer deaths, according to the US Department of Health and Human Services, is estimated to be about 30 percent. This means that we can expect that 129,000 Americans will die of cancer this year because of the higher overall cancer rate that exists among smokers as compared to nonsmokers.

In fact, cigarette smokers have a total cancer death rate

two times greater than do nonsmokers. And there is no single action any individual can take to reduce the risk of cancer more effectively than giving up cigarettes.

It might sound like a simple solution to a complex problem. But despite the overwhelming scientific evidence on the health hazards of smoking, smokers seem willing to take their chances, puffing away at an estimated 615 billion cigarettes each year.

The diseases associated with smoking are numerous, from lung cancer to heart ailments. There are other dangers as well. Mothers who smoke during pregnancy, for example, increase the risk of spontaneous abortion. Babies born to women who smoke during pregnancy are on the average seven ounces lighter than babies born to women who don't smoke. And there is strong evidence to suggest that the average young male smoker (thirty to forty years old) who smokes more than forty cigarettes per day loses an estimated eight years of life.

Is it then any wonder that smoking is considered the number-one public health enemy in America?

The decision to quit smoking may not only extend your life, but save it as well. Government studies, for example, show that the death rate for male cigarette smokers—irrespective of how much they smoked—is much higher than for nonsmoking males. Also, death rates are higher for smokers who began at a younger age compared to people who began smoking later in life.

Of course, as you learned in the previous chapter, the longer you remain smokeless the less risk you run of expiring from a tobacco-related illness. In fact, after fifteen years of remaining smoke-free, mortality rates for the former smoker are similar to those of people who never smoked at all.

Let's continue to examine the havoc that puff of tobacco smoke wreaks on your body. For example, in just three seconds after you inhale its smoke, a cigarette makes your heart beat faster, increases your blood pressure, and substitutes deadly carbon monoxide for the oxygen in your bloodstream. In this short amount of time smoke coursing through your body already leaves cancer-causing chemicals to be absorbed by your organs. The more you smoke, the more of these dangerous chemicals are left behind.

Smoking also narrows the blood vessels that carry blood to the skin—especially the fingers and toes. And if you are suffering from any form of heart disease, constricted blood vessels complicate the situation by forcing the heart to pump harder. Those cigarettes are also causing great harm to your lungs. The tar, carbon monoxide, and hydrogen cyanide all found in cigarette smoke damage the lung tissue. Scientists are also finding, for example, that carbon monoxide interferes with blood cells which transport oxygen, and can result in premature aging.

The extraordinary serious health consequences of smoking, as we previously pointed out, just don't seem to deter people from smoking. This despite the fact that in one government study 70 to 80 percent of smokers who were interviewed agreed that cigarettes are harmful, are a dangerous health hazard, and can cause disease and death. In that same study, former and new ex-smokers like yourself took a much stronger stand on these issues.

The trend is a disturbing one. In 1915 only about 18 billion cigarettes were consumed annually as compared to the more than 600 billion that are smoked today. Scientists became suspicious of cigarettes as a cause of illness and death as early as the 1930s, because of an increase in the lung cancer rate. In the 1930s, less than 3,000 Americans were listed as dying of this disease. By the 1950's, that figure had grown to 18,000 annually. Today, some estimates are as high as 100,000 deaths each year from lung cancer.

All this is not to say that people don't try to quit smoking— they do. According to government figures, approximately 60

Annual Death Rates of Smokers Broken Down by Various Factors
(Rates given per 100,000 people)

By Inhalation Pattern				
	Degree of Inhalation			
Age	*None*	*Slight*	*Moderate*	*Deep*
45–54	824	859	974	1,021
55–64	1,868	2,376	2,351	2,689
65–74	3,994	5,029	5,300	6,411

By Age at Onset of Smoking					
	Age Began Smoking				
Age	*Under 14*	*15–19*	*20–24*	*25–29*	*30+*
45–54	1,210	999	857	726	562
55–64	2,682	2,509	2,058	2,082	1,576
65–74	6,221	5,728	4,728	3,902	3,846

By Number of Cigarettes Smoked Daily				
	Number of Cigarettes			
Sex and Age	*1–9*	*10–19*	*20–39*	*40+*
Males				
45–54	741	910	970	1,109
55–64	1,815	2,280	2,437	2,680
65–74	4,683	5,145	5,325	5,635
Females				
45–54	288	368	464	592
55–64	682	904	1,010	Insufficient data
65–74	2,055	2,238	2,862	Insufficient data

Source: US Department of Health and Human Services.

percent of the more than 50 million current adult smokers in this country have tried to stop smoking at one time or another. These figures also indicate that within any given year, more young people between the ages of seventeen and twenty-four try to quit than their elders.

In one recent study of smokers, nine out of ten people interviewed said that they had either tried to stop smoking or would do so if there were an easy method they could use. At the same time, approximately 95 percent of former smokers who did break the habit said they were able to do so on their own with no assistance. They credited determination as the motivating force which kept them smokeless.

Researchers say another trend has developed among the nation's smoking population since 1965 which offers a glimmer of hope in a rather gloomy situation. According to government studies, there has been a decline in adult smoking of approximately 42 percent since that year.

It is a hopeful indication that more and more people are breaking the yoke of nicotine addiction. Perhaps smokers are finally coming to their senses in not wanting to play Russian roulette with their lives. None of us needs to let smoke get in our eyes . . .

Tobacco Road

A cigarette may look harmless enough, but it is a dangerous nesting ground of poisonous gases and chemical substances. According to researchers, tobacco and tobacco smoke contain more than 1,200 clearly identified substances in addition to millions of particulates, or minute separate particles, which break down and recombine to form new compounds.

Such harmful substances include tar, carbon monoxide,

nicotine, arsenic, trioxide, nickel carbonyl, acrolein, phenol, ammonia, a radioactive chemical called potassium 210, prussic acid, strychnine, formaldehyde, pyrene, and other compounds.

The following is a brief description of some of the more dangerous substances found in tobacco and tobacco smoke:

Tar: Think of that smelly, gooey stuff used by street repaving crews and you'll get the idea. Tar is a mass of particulate matter. When you inhale, tiny droplets glue themselves to your mouth, throat and lungs. Tar can cause cancer.

Carbon Monoxide: This is a colorless, odorless, and very poisonous gas. It poisons the healthy red blood cells in your body. Many people have died while sitting in an unventilated car with the engine running and giving off carbon monoxide fumes.

Formaldehyde: This is the fluid used to embalm dead bodies. It is a colorless, irritating gas present in cigarette smoke.

Ammonia: Did you ever have to turn your head after opening a bottle of ammonia? In the body it irritates delicate membranes in the nose and throat. It also causes destruction of lung tissue when inhaled deeply.

Strychnine: A deadly poison.

Arsenic: Ditto.

Cadmium: A poisonous metallic element that is suspected of causing emphysema.

Hydrogen cyanide: A poisonous compound used in gas chambers.

Acrolein: Poisonous to cilia in the body. Can cause cancer when combined with other compounds.

Phenol: Same as above.

Just how deadly is continued exposure to cigarette smoke? Researchers believe that such exposure can lead to serious health problems. The following tables, compiled by government researchers, indicate the major toxic agents in the gases and particles found in tobacco smoke.

Gases		Particulates	
Dimethylnitrosamine	C*	Benzopyrene	TI
Ethylmethylnitrosamine	C	5-Methylchrysene	TI
Diethylnitrosamine	C	Benzofluoranthene	TI
Nitrosopyrrolidine	C	Benzanthracene	TI
Hydrazine	C	Dibenzacridine	TI
Vinyl chloride	C	Pyrene	C
Urethane	TI	Fluoranthene	C
Formaldehyde	C	Benzo perylene	C
Hydrogen cyanide	T	Naphthalenes	C
Acrolein	T	Polonium-210	C
Acetaldehyde	T	Nickel compounds	C
Nitrogen oxides	T	Cadmium compounds	C
Carbon monoxide	T	Arsenic	C
		Nicotine	T
		Minor tobacco alkaloids	T
		Phenol	T
		Cresols	T

* C: cancer causing; TI: tumor initiator; T: toxic.

Nicotine: The Nature of the Beast

Okay, so far we've talked about withdrawal and some of the hazards of smoking. But we really haven't met the beast yet—that incredibly powerful poison called nicotine.

Nicotine is, in fact, so powerful that it can be downright lethal. A dosage of sixty milligrams can kill as quickly as cyanide. Such a dosage would at first cause the nausea and dizziness experienced by beginning smokers and ultimately result in convulsions and respiratory failure.

You might say that sixty milligrams is more nicotine than most average smokers will ingest. Wrong. That's the actual amount of nicotine contained in about two packs of cigarettes. When you think about it—and we have—a pack-a-day smoker inhales about 7,300 milligrams of nicotine in a year. The only reason why we don't have a glut of coronor's reports that read "death by nicotine poisoning" is that the smoker consumes this alkaloid poison in small amounts—one cigarette at a time—so that the body can absorb and metabolize it without instantly serious harmful effects.

Scientists have also found that smokers unconsciously vary their inhalation rate, thus keeping the nicotine levels in their bloodstream at a fairly constant level. It is when that level drops that the smoker has the proverbial "nicotine fit" and reaches for another smoke. With that first puff, the nicotine level in the bloodstream is quickly restored. It is a fast-acting process. Nicotine inhaled from a cigarette actually reaches the brain in about seven seconds flat—twice as fast as if you had injected that same amount of nicotine into your arm.

In general terms, between 15 and 25 percent of the nicotine in tobacco is inhaled in what is called "mainstream" smoke (that concentrated drag which travels the length of the cigarette and is inhaled). About 90 percent of this "mainstream" smoke is absorbed by the lungs. It enters the lung capillaries and from there scoots up to the brain via the arteries.

That shot of nicotine does a lot of things to your body. It increases the secretion of saliva and inhibits stomach contractions and causes all the other physiologic changes we discussed earlier in this chapter. In short, it causes chaos in your insides.

Nicotine is a deceptive beast. What smoker, after all, hasn't claimed that smoking has a relaxing effect. Of course, we know the opposite is true. Nicotine constricts blood vessels, raises your blood pressure, makes the heart beat faster, and causes an overall condition that more closely resembles stress than relaxation.

But this is only a brief introduction to the beast. We'll be meeting him again and again throughout the pages of this book. Let's make a brief digression and then return to our study of the subject at hand.

T·H·R·E·E

THE BODY ECLECTIC

Let's talk for a few minutes about calories before returning to our discussion of nicotine and its effects on the body. For the new ex-smoker, calories are the stuff that nightmares are made of—so let's see how they work.

Most people don't know this, but smokers usually weigh less than nonsmokers. In fact, smokers weigh an average of about seven pounds less than their smokeless counterparts. The question, of course, is: Why?

There is no definitive answer to this question, but some researchers believe that nicotine may be the cause of this weight differential. One theory has it that nicotine alters the process of digestion. The digestive process is so affected that smokers are *less able* to efficiently store the calories they take in with their meals. The result, of course, is a thinner you.

Nonsmokers, on the other hand, are *more* efficiently able to store those calories. So if they take in more of them than they expend during the day's activities, the result is weight gain.

For example, as you sit and read this book you're using up about 80 calories an hour. If you're munching a bag of potato chips at the same time (about 120 calories), you're taking in 40 more calories than you're expending.

This is an important figure, because your body counts calories much more efficiently than you do. If it receives more than it requires, the body will simply turn such excess calories into fat and store them. This is nature's way of insuring that if we don't eat, there still will be an energy supply handy to keep our vital body organs functioning.

A smoker, however, does not store some of those extra calories. Through a peculiar digestive process, the mechanics of which are still not clearly known, the body sloughs off these calories that would otherwise be stored as fat. He or she thus remains thinner than the nonsmoker—unnaturally so.

All right, now let's return to our discussion of nicotine and see what influence it exerts on altering the normal process of metabolism.

Metabolism is nothing more than the *rate* at which your body uses calories. Let's again consider the example of the 80 calories per hour you're using to read this book. If you put the book down and decide to take a nap, you'll be using even fewer calories. The amount of calories your body is burning up in this resting state is called the basal metabolic rate, or BMR.

Everyone does not have the same BMR. It varies considerably with each individual. People who are of the same age, sex, and weight may differ in their BMR by as much as 30 percent. Age is an important factor in metabolism, because as you grow older your metabolic rate slows down.

For example, a twelve-year-old boy's average BMR may be 50. In other words, he's using 50 calories an hour just to rest. At age forty-nine, that now-grown boy's metabolism has slowed down to about 40. He's now using 40 calories to rest.

Let's suppose our forty-nine-year-old man is typical of many adult males his age—he's probably still eating about as much as he did when he was twelve. If that's the case, he's going to have a problem common to many middle-aged people— obesity.

Why? Because the higher one's metabolic rate, the more calories one burns up while engaged in any physical activity. Consequently, a person with a higher BMR may eat more than one with a slower metabolism.

Nicotine, interestingly enough, seems to *increase* the metabolic rate, which means that a smoker is burning off more calories doing exactly the same thing as a nonsmoker! Yet popular wisdom continues to maintain that the reason why smokers are thinner than nonsmokers is because they eat less.

Not true, at least according to some of the latest research on the subject. In fact, researchers are proving just the opposite—that in many cases, smokers actually eat *more* than nonsmokers but remain slimmer because of the effects of nicotine.

A recent study conducted with male cigarette smokers indicated that they consumed about 350 calories a day more than nonsmokers in the study group. Yet the smokers remained thinner than the nonsmokers. If you were—or are—a heavy smoker, chances are you consume as much as 575 more calories per day than nonsmokers. That's like eating a whole extra meal!

But as a smoker, you probably didn't consume all those extra calories in one sitting. Instead, you tended to not only eat more food at regular meals than nonsmokers, but also consumed more snacks and alcoholic beverages to go along with your smoking habit. After all, beer, snacks, and cigarettes go together as naturally as cream-cheese, bagels, and lox. Unfair as it might have seemed to your more diet-conscious, nonsmoking friends, you still weighed an average of seven pounds less than they did.

If smokers can eat more and not gain weight, do former smokers retain the same advantage? Unfortunately, no. Research indicates pretty conclusively that when we give up cigarettes most of us will *gain* weight. Also, there seems to be a direct link between how much you used to smoke and the amount you will gain as an ex-smoker. The sad fact is that the more heavily you smoked, the more pounds you'll tend to add after quitting. This could also be related to the effects of metabolism, but current research on the subject is still scant.

What the latest research does clearly indicate, however, is that after just a few months of not smoking, the average ex-smoker has gained about 8 pounds. In a five-year study on 501 telephone installers and repairmen who stopped smoking, seven out of eight men gained an average of 4 pounds. One unfortunate fellow put on an incredible 114 pounds.

Why do we gain weight after quitting the habit? To answer that question it's important to understand some of the physical changes that are occurring in our bodies after we snuff out that last cigarette.

About a week after we've tossed our last package of cigarettes into the garbage, our metabolism and digestion have been liberated from the effects of nicotine. Our body is returning to normal. Our metabolism is now slowing down and we are beginning to more efficiently store those calories we used to slough off when we smoked. Unfortunately, this means if we eat exactly the same way we did as smokers, weight gain is inevitable.

Okay, so far so bad. But to make matters worse, we may even be unconsciously changing our eating patterns and preferences in ways that make us gain more weight.

Why should going smokeless change our eating habits? Once again, our old enemy, nicotine, enters the picture. Research has shown that when experimental nicotine-addicted animals are no longer administered nicotine, they eat more sugar—*not greater amounts of all foods.* In another study, habitual smokers were not allowed to smoke during one session and could smoke freely at the next. The subjects were provided with a variety of foods. When not smoking, those who participated in the study consumed roughly twice as much sweet and salty foods as they did while smoking.

The results seem to indicate that the sweets were simply a substitute for smoking. Thus it's also possible that an ex-smoker may begin to use certain foods in a similar manner—as a substitute for that cigarette so sorely missed.

Before we continue along this line of investigation, let's first backtrack a bit and take a closer look at what prompted us to reach for that package of cigarettes in the first place.

By and large, it was a pretty automatic gesture. We didn't very often consciously inform ourselves that we were going to light up. We just reached for a cigarette and did it! If, as former smokers, we're now substituting certain foods for cigarettes, chances are this kind of eating is also being done on the subconscious level.

But even such unconscious habits as smoking, overeating, or noshing on the wrong stuff do not function in and of themselves. They require a cue or trigger. Those "triggers" can be divided into two categories: the emotional and the physical. Emotional triggers can be described as feelings or moods. Boredom, stress, and happiness are just three of many. Physical triggers can be such things as watching television or ending a meal.

If there is one universal "trigger" for smokers, it is the end of a meal. Every smoker lights up when he or she is finished eating—it's just a question of how quickly they reach for that cigarette. It is that satisfying moment—a sort of ritual of completion. When you quit smoking, that signal which marks the end of a meal is lost. As a result, the ex-smoker may just continue eating. Now you may be marking the end of a meal by your absolute inability to eat any more.

Right about now, based upon what you've read so far, you're probably thinking that it makes a lot more sense to resume smoking if you're at all concerned about your weight. The truth of the matter is, however, that you would have to gain more than *seventy-five pounds* to offset the health benefits you've derived by breaking the habit. That, nonetheless, may be small consolation if you are watching with some dismay your growing waistline.

But hold on a second! Are we really doomed to accept weight gain as a natural but inevitable consequence of giving up smoking? Fortunately, the answer to that question is a definite no.

Let's now suppose you're a new ex-smoker who regrettably has begun to put on a few pounds. The first thing to avoid is becoming angry, frustrated, or panicky. Instead, try to find out exactly what is causing such weight gain.

You may have discovered as an ex-smoker that the solution to ridding yourself of those excess pounds is not as simple as reaching for the latest crash diet book (more on such "miracle" diets later). And we can tell you right now that there's much more involved in losing weight than simply trying to eliminate those pancakes filled with jam, sugar, and cinnamon—although it's a good start. Not only do each of us have unique weight problems when we give up cigarettes, but we must deal with those problems on an individual basis. It's going to take some effort, but you've come this far already!

Many "quit smoking" clinics encourage their clients to analyze their smoking patterns. That is a good idea. The theory behind this is that only after you know what your smoking patterns are can you begin to modify your behavior. Awareness, in fact, is one of the key principles upon which such behavior modification is based. As we have discussed earlier, just as you had individual smoking patterns, so do you have individual eating habits which may have changed as a result of your not smoking without your even realizing it.

Are you, for example, substituting more food and certain kinds of foods for cigarettes? Have you increased your consumption of sweets? Or is your weight gain simply the product of metabolic changes within your body?

One way to determine your individual eating patterns and take that important first step toward formulating your individual program for weight control is to keep a record of everything you've eaten for at least a week. Keep this "Food-Intake Record" along with your "Emotions Chart" on page 42. After a week or so, you'll have a much clearer idea of what you are eating, why you are eating certain foods, and when and how you are eating.

While you're compiling this record, let's reserve judgment on what effects your eating habits are having on your weight. For the time being, let's again turn to the role of metabolism in the ex-smoker's battle of the bulge.

FOOD-INTAKE RECORD

Time of Day	Type of Food	Place	Mood or Reason for Eating
1.			
2.			
3.			
4.			
5.			
6.			
7.			
8.			

9. _____

10. _____

11. _____

12. _____

13. _____

14. _____

15. _____

16. _____

17. _____

18. _____

19. _____

20. _____

F · O · U · R

THE DOUBLE WHAMMY

You may recall reading in the previous chapter that the new ex-smoker gains an average of about eight pounds in a few months. What we didn't tell you is that those pounds can accumulate even if daily caloric consumption is cut by as much as 200 calories!

In fact, a drastic cut in your caloric intake may be the worst possible step in your battle against the bulge. Alas, that seems to be the first reaction by many former smokers who observe with some alarm the relentless slide upward of the needle on the bathroom scale.

Unbeknownst to the new dieter, a sharp reduction in calories mobilizes the body's defensive reaction to dieting. Any sudden decrease in food intake causes the body to decrease its energy output. Why? Because our body is an expert when it comes to energy conservation. Any large cut in calories signals less incoming fuel, so conservation measures are put into effect. Metabolism slows down and other reactions take place to make certain that the functioning of vital organs is not impaired.

The brain initiates a red alert. Defense systems go into effect. Your body, fearful you may starve to death, refuses to waste any more calories. Our hapless ex-smoker is now confronted with a unique dilemma—what we call the "double whammy." Not only has his or her metabolism slowed down somewhat in response to going smokeless, but it is slowing down even further to counteract the effects of crash dieting. The end result of all this is the body's stubborn refusal to lose any more weight. It's a Mexican standoff, even if your caloric intake remains the same.

Again you are probably thinking that perhaps it was a mistake, after all, to join the smoke-free generation. But take heart. This is not the end of the line. We'll get you back in shape, yet. But, first, let's backtrack a bit and take a look at the weighty problem of obesity without the added complication of giving up cigarettes.

We all know that overweight people "pig out" more than their thinner peers, right? After all, that's why they're so fat in the first place. Well, perhaps not so. New research suggests that in many cases obese individuals *do not* eat more than skinnier people. In some cases, researchers found that they actually *ate less*.

A recent study conducted with 500 pairs of middle-aged brothers—with one of the pair living in Boston and the other in Ireland—found that those brothers who lived in the United States ate less than their Irish relatives but weighed more. The study determined that the Irish side of the family was far more active than their American counterparts.

In other words, the amount and kind of physical activity can tip the scale to either thin or fat. Even moderate physical activity raises your metabolic rate, and any activity which lifts your BMR above its resting stage results in increased caloric expenditure—and that means you shed pounds.

Of course, the amount of calories one expends is entirely dependent on the type, duration, and intensity of the activity. *Exercise is the key that unlocks every door to weight control.* It can keep the new ex-smoker from gaining weight, and, if you've already added those excess pounds, exercise can help you lose them. In fact, a program of physical exercise can actually compensate for the metabolic slowdown caused by both quitting smoking and dieting!

Exercise for Weight Loss and Keeping It Off

Right about now, in addition to catching our breath after all this talk about exercise, it would also be terrific if we could recommend a standardized program of physical exercise for all new nonsmokers or those seriously thinking about quitting. But that's too much like trying to recommend a generic diet. Exercise programs and diets should be catered to your individual needs.

One of the best ways to begin *your* exercise program is to first pick an activity that you enjoy doing. If you like a particular exercise, you'll be far more likely to stick with it. But let's face it. Even if you basically enjoy that activity, at first you're going to have to use willpower to maintain the regimen. But if there's one thing we ex-smokers know about ourselves, it's that we have plenty of willpower!

Beginning an exercise program won't take the monumental amount of inner fortitude it did to put out that last cigarette. In time, we predict that you'll actually come to enjoy your new active lifestyle—so much so, that you wouldn't dream of going back to your old, more sedate ways.

Many "quit smoking" programs emphasize visual reminders not to smoke, such as a written contract or a 12-month calendar with each month checked off for not smoking. You might try the same thing with your exercise program. Such a daily chart would list the miles you walked or bicycled, the distances you swam or jogged. That exercise record, like your no-smoking record, is really something to be proud of!

The best kind of physical activity for both fitness and weight control should include some form of aerobic exercise. One of the most popular forms of this exercise is aerobic dance. However, any type of activity in which there is constant motion from fifteen to forty minutes at a heart rate of 120 to 150 beats per minute is considered aerobic. Swimming, cycling, jogging, walking—even skipping rope—all fit into this category.

Nonaerobic or anaerobic sports are stop/start sports such as tennis, badminton, volleyball, and bowling. These are short-duration, straining exercises that pump little oxygen into the bloodstream. Such activities are especially good for developing coordination and muscle strength, but less effective for cardiovascular improvement or weight loss.

The good news for the new nonsmoker is that aerobic exercise has the opposite effect of smoking on the body. Whereas smoking robs the body of its ability to absorb and distribute oxygen, aerobic exercises promote both these functions.

In the fitness revolution that is sweeping America, aerobic exercises seem to be the people's choice because they are efficient calorie busters, can be done with others, require a minimal amount of equipment, and do not produce a high injury rate. Aerobic exercises are also an easily available form of exercise.

Again, as is the case with any type of exercise program you may want to get involved with, the key words are *frequency, duration,* and *intensity.* It is also important to first seek the guidance of a physician before undertaking any prolonged strenuous activity. Otherwise you could risk suffering undue pain, discomfort, or something even more serious.

FREQUENCY— Most experts seem to agree that if total fitness is your primary objective, you should exercise three days a week with a day of rest between workouts. There is, to date, no conclusive evidence to indicate that by exercising every day you become fitter. On the other hand, if as a new ex-smoker your goal is to work off those extra pounds or maintain your present weight, it is advisable to try and exercise five or six days a week, because the more you work out the greater number of calories you will burn up.

DURATION— Even a three-to-five-minute spurt of vigorous exercise performed three times a week will improve your aerobic fitness level and take off some weight. However, your best bet is to undertake a less strenuous regimen for twenty minutes or longer on three separate days. This method will not only improve the pumping ability of your heart, but also enhance the body's ability to absorb and consume oxygen. As a result, you will soon be able to exercise every day in order to lose weight, and not feel fatigued. And, as we've just noted, the more you exercise the thinner you get.

INTENSITY— The rule of thumb is that, whatever physical activity you may be involved in, it should be strenuous enough to produce a heartbeat rate that is between 60 and 75 percent of your maximum heartbeat rate—and that this rate be sustained for at least fifteen minutes. When we talk about maximum heart rates, we mean the fastest that your heart is capable of beating while exercising. Don't start out your exercise program by pushing the limit. Strive for the 60-percent target zone (see chart, p. 73) and keep it there for the first few months. As you get into better and better shape, shoot for the 75-percent level.

Although some people—especially athletes—can raise their

target rate to 85 percent or higher after months of exercise, you do not have to work that hard to stay in good condition. In fact, studies by the National Institutes of Mental Health have demonstrated that there is no special benefit to be derived by exceeding the 75-percent target zone. You might also keep in mind that if you enjoy certain nonaerobic sports such as downhill skiing, you need not avoid them. As the chart at the conclusion of this chapter indicates, even a vigorous game of handball, raquetball, or squash can burn off calories if played briskly for at least thirty minutes.

We've talked a bit about maximum heart rates and target zones, so now it's time for you to learn how to establish your own target zone during exercise. Your maximum heart rate during brisk activity is usually 220 beats per minute minus your age. If, for example, you are twenty years old, your maximum heart rate is approximately 200. If you consult the chart we've provided you with in this chapter, you will find that your 60-to-75-percent range during exercise should average out to between 120 and 150 beats per minute. But because it is important that you monitor your heart rate ten seconds after doing five minutes of exercise (your heart rate begins to drop about ten seconds after the cessation of exercise), we have provided you with a second chart on pg. 74 that will help you find your target zone within this time frame.

Try to remain within your target zone. If, for example, at age twenty your ten-second heart rate averages out to 28, you are too far out of the safe zone, so slow down. If your pulse shows a heart rate of 20, you're getting insufficient aerobic benefit, so increase your pace. Above all, try to use common sense. As a former smoker, it is unlikely that you have engaged in any strenuous exercise for some time, so take it easy. No matter how slowly you begin, you'll feel more fit after a few weeks of exercise than when you first started.

You now know how to figure out your target zone, but

some of you may not know how to take your pulse to determine at what rate your heart is beating. Here is how to do so:

1. While exercising, wear a watch with a moving second hand. If you are swimming, most pool clocks have second hands.
2. Turn your right hand palm up.
3. Place the tips of the fingers of your left hand on your right wrist.
4. Find the bone of your wrist under the right thumb where the wrist and the hand join.
5. Move the tips of your fingers a bit to the left and press firmly with the index, middle, and ring fingers. You should feel a pulse.
6. If you're having problems, put the index finger of your right hand under the left jawbone and over one of the large blood vessels on your neck (the carotid arteries). You should feel a strong pulse.
7. Take your pulse ten seconds after the cessation of exercise—ideally after about five minutes of exercise.

Physical Activity Programs

As a former smoker now involving yourself in a physical activity program, you are joining more than half the United States population who are doing the same. According to a recent survey conducted by the President's Council on Physical Fitness and Sports, more than 55 percent of adult Americans—some 60 million people—engage in some form of exercise. Of those 60 million, it is estimated that 44 million Americans exercise by walking, 18 million bicycle regularly, 14 million swim, and 6.5 million Americans jog. An estimated 14 million Americans do some type of calisthenics and many people in this country participate in more than one form of exercise.

So, welcome to the club. And remember that, if losing pounds is why you are going to involve yourself in regular physical activity, you should stick to a program which lasts a minimum of twenty minutes per day for a maximum of six days a week. Your long-range goal is to work off at least 300 calories at each exercise session.

The following table indicates the number of calories that are burned up per hour for a given aerobic exercise. Source is the National Institute of Public Health.

Bicycling (6 mph)	240 cal
Bicycling (12 mph)	410 cal
Cross-country skiing (per hour)	700 cal
Jogging (5½ mph)	660 cal
Jogging (7 mph)	920 cal
Jumping rope (per hour)	750 cal
Running in place (per hour)	650 cal
Running (10 mph)	1,280 cal
Swimming (25 yds/min for 1 hour)	275 cal
Swimming (50 yds/min for 1 hour)	500 cal
Walking (2 mph)	240 cal
Walking (3 mph)	320 cal
Walking (4½ mph)	440 cal

(Note: The calories spent in a particular activity vary in proportion to body weight.)

The following table indicates the approximate number of calories that are burned up per hour for a given anaerobic exercise. Source is the US Department of Health and Human Services.

Racquetball (sustained)	675 cal
Bowling	220 cal
Canoeing (4 mph)	401 cal
Volleyball	220–450 cal
Rowboating (2½ mph)	300 cal
Golf	245 cal
Badminton	350 cal
Handball (sustained)	591 cal
Calisthenics	300–360 cal
Ice skating (10 mph)	360–420 cal
Fencing	300 cal
Square dancing	350 cal
Gardening	220 cal
Tennis	400 cal

The following figures are averages and should be used as general guidelines in determining your safe heart rate during exercise. Look for the age category closest to your age and read the line across. The maximum heart rate is usually 220 minus your age. Source is the National Institutes of Health.

Age	Target Zone (60–75 percent)	Average Maximum Heart Rate (100 percent)
20 years	120–150 beats/min	200
25 years	117–146 beats/min	195
30 years	114–142 beats/min	190
35 years	111–138 beats/min	185
40 years	108–135 beats/min	180
45 years	105–131 beats/min	175
50 years	102–127 beats/min	170
55 years	99–123 beats/min	165
60 years	96–120 beats/min	160
65 years	93–116 beats/min	155
70 years	90–113 beats/min	150

This table indicates how quickly your heart will pump blood under conditions of brisk exercise. It is to be used as a general guideline to determine what the safe ten-second pulse rate should be after cessation of exercise. Source is National Institutes of Health.

Age	Ten-Second Target Rate
20	25
25	24
30	24
35	24
40	24
45	23
50	23
55	23
60	23
65	22
70	22

F · I · V · E

THESE BOOTS ARE MADE
FOR WALKING

Whether you walk, run, jog, cycle or belly dance, exercise is the name of the game in any weight-control program you may decide to embark upon.

The key to effective weight control is keeping energy intake (food) and activity output in balance. Weight depends not only on how many calories are taken in during the day, but also how many are used up in an exercise program.

There are probably as many misconceptions about exercising as there are about dieting. One very popular myth which seeks to debunk the value of exercise holds that it increases your appetite. This argument holds that after an hour of swimming, jogging or whatever, you become ravenously hungry—so hungry, in fact, that you rush right home and eat twice the amount you would have if you did not exercise. According to this line of reasoning, such an eating binge cancels out all that exercising has accomplished. Actually, most studies done on the subject indicate that there is a small *lowering* of food consumption unless the activity is a very strenuous one such as football. While it is true that a lean person in good condition may eat more following increased activity, his exercise will burn up the extra calories he or she consumes.

Laboratory tests on experimental animals have borne this out. When their exercise was moderate, food intake did not increase. In one experiment animals that exercised one hour a day actually ate a smaller amount of food than those that exercised less than one hour a day or not at all! On the other hand, when the animals were exercised vigorously over longer periods, they ate more, but the extra activity kept their weight constant.

In other experiments, when the animals' activity was decreased, if they continued to eat the same amount of food they became obese. Similarly, a study of overweight adults showed that the start of their obesity corresponded with their decline in activity. Although their activity decreased, their appetites didn't.

Another popular argument against exercise is that by only ridding the body of 300 calories per exercise session, "It's going to take me forever to lose that weight—so why should I bother?" To answer that, we need only to borrow some long-lasting and sagacious advice from the ancient Chinese: "A journey of a thousand miles begins with one step." The important thing here is to *keep moving!*

Consistency is the key to exercising. If a person only expends 75 to 100 calories per day in a twenty-minute walk, that same person would lose ten pounds in a year. Most importantly, the latest scientific research strongly suggests that exercise produces an increase in metabolic rate that *actually outlasts the activity.* Even light exercise reportedly produces a post-activity increase in metabolism equivalent to sloughing off between 40 and 50 extra calories. Really strenuous exercise, like football or rugby, burns off an additional 450 calories in the aftermath of the game. The point is that just by doing some none-too-strenuous exercise—like walking—you're getting a 50-calorie bonus per session. So that lunchtime walk, in which you're trying to work off a goal of 300 calories, really means that you're burning off 350 calories.

Before we outline some aerobic activities you might want to get involved in, a few pointers might be in order on how to maximize your success with a new physical fitness program:

Remember to think of your exercise program as fun. Begin slowly. You don't have to start jogging or running a mile your first few days out; instead run or jog a block, then two blocks, etc. If you're going to ride a bicycle in order to lose or maintain weight, start off at two miles a day and gradually pedal your way up to six miles. In other words, set your sights on short-term as well as long-term goals.

Discuss your exercise program and goals with your family and friends. Their encouragement and understanding are important sources of support that can help you keep going. They may even want to join in.

Variety always helps to make any exercise enjoyable. Repetition can become deadly. For example, instead of jogging continuously around a track, why not jog for a few minutes, then run—even skip or hop—around the track for a while? If you plan to swim, don't just do laps. Vary your strokes. That way you'll work out all parts of your body.

If you're feeling bored or aren't enjoying a particular activity, then try a different conditioning exercise. Try to establish certain hours during the day for your fitness program. Some people prefer mornings because they claim exercise energizes them for the remainder of the day. Others like to work out after work, arguing that it relieves them of the stresses of the day.

Whatever time of day or night you choose for your activity,

make sure that you dress comfortably. And always warm up before an exercise—five to ten minutes of low-intensity movements are recommended. And always remember that you should cool down after completing a workout. Again, five to ten minutes of low-level exercise combined with some stretching are recommended.

Try to work out with a friend or in a small group. It's much more enjoyable to exercise when you have company, which is why health clubs are so popular in this country. Friends also help to motivate you.

Try to keep a record of your progress. And when you attain a short-range or long-range goal, reward yourself. One good way to motivate yourself is to work out a system of such rewards before you get involved in a fitness or weight-loss activity program.

We've emphasized the importance of warming up before you exercise and cooling down afterward. The following are a few stretching exercises that should be done slowly and in a steady, rhythmical way. Your exercise session should last anywhere from twenty minutes to an hour. An ideal time is twenty-five to forty minutes and should include a five-minute warm-up, fifteen to thirty minutes of exercising within your target zone, and a five-minute cool-down.

Okay, first some warm-up exercises:

WALL PUSH—Stand about 1½ feet away from the wall. Then lean forward pushing against the wall, keeping heels flat. Count to ten then rest. Repeat one to two times.

PALM TOUCH—Stand with your knees slightly bent. Then bend from the waist and try to touch your palms to the floor. Do not bounce. Count to ten then rest. Repeat one to two times. If you have lower back problems, do this exercise with your legs crossed.

TOE TOUCH—Place your right leg level on a stair, chair, or other object. Keeping your other leg straight, lean forward and slowly try to touch your right toe. Do this with your right hand ten times and with your left hand ten times. Then switch legs and repeat with each hand. Repeat entire exercise one to two times.

To cool down after exercising simply slow down gradually. For example, swim more slowly or change to a more leisurely stroke. If you've been running, walk briskly. If you're through riding a bicycle, get off and walk with it for a while. If you've been jogging, running, or walking briskly, you might want to repeat some of your stretching and limbering exercises to loosen up your muscles. We will offer a few specific exercises for joggers and runners a bit later in this chapter.

Right now, let's get into a couple of aerobic activities that are solid choices when you're exercising for weight loss.

Bicycling

The origin of the bicycle dates back to 2300 B.C., a fact you may want to keep handy the next time you play a game of Trivial Pursuit. It was thought about, at least on paper, in ancient China, and later in ancient Egypt and India, but never built.

The French were to claim that accomplishment. It was a Frenchman—Count Mede de Sivrac—who, in 1790, built what is thought to be the world's first bicycle. This prototype had two wheels linked by a narrow wood bridge and was driven by alternate pushes of the feet on the ground.

Frenchmen fell in love with this mode of transportation, and two years later had perfected the state of the art so that they could pedal about at speeds up to fifteen kilometers per hour.

The fad spread throughout the world, and modification of bicycle construction—as of cars—never ceased. In 1932 the first gear-changing system was introduced at the world road racing championships.

Today the bicycle is used not only by serious road riders involved in a variety of competitions, but by everyone from the age of eight to eighty. It's a fun form of exercise, is aerobically beneficial, and, for us new ex-smokers, bicycling helps get us in gear for our weight-control program.

If you are planning to bicycle outdoors—as opposed to using an indoor exercycle—make certain your bike has a speedometer as well as an odometer, a device which measures the distance traveled. As with any other aerobic activity you might engage in, you should do some warm-up exercises before you begin. Some sit-ups to strengthen your back muscles, a couple of push-ups for handlebar muscles, and a few of the stretching exercises described earlier will do nicely. A little in-place jogging and a few jumping jacks to work up some sweat is also recommended.

Now you're ready to begin. Remember, start off easy. A speed of fifty-five to sixty revolutions per minute is just fine for the first ten minutes of your ride. Then move up to the seventy to eighty rpm speed and check to make sure your heart rate is within its elevated target range.

A program suggested for the new ex-smoker is that he or she begin a regimen at two miles per day for five days a week. Your time goal should be between twelve and fourteen minutes. If you're more than fifty years old, however, take thirteen to sixteen minutes to reach this goal. Keep increasing your distance one mile every three weeks. Your long-range goal is to get on that bicycle and do six miles in approximately thirty minutes.

Whether you are striving for a short-range or long-range goal in your program, just remember to keep your legs going all the time with no coasting. And if you're just beginning, avoid pedaling up hills because it will wear you out too quickly. When you complete your ride, get off your bike and walk around a while until your pulse rate returns to normal. If you stop cold, you will stiffen up. This is also a good time to do a few more of those stretching exercises.

All right, you'd rather watch "General Hospital" while cycling instead of checking out the local scenery—especially on super-hot or cold days. Fine. There's absolutely nothing wrong with pedaling off those calories on an exercycle.

When you purchase an exercycle—and some models sell for as little as forty dollars—make sure it has a speedometer, odometer, and controls for tension adjustment and seat adjustment.

For the indoor cyclist, duration rather than distance is the key, because you won't be traveling far on this stationary piece of equipment. Make sure your seat is adjusted so that one knee is almost straight down in the pedal position. Okay, now turn on the television set and we're ready to go for a spin.

A good way to begin your program is to pedal ten miles per hour for five minutes. Try to raise your heart rate to at least 125 beats per minute if you're less than fifty years old. If you're older than that, your elevated heart rate should be a minimum of 100 to 110 beats per minute. At this age, cycle for four minutes rather than five.

Your long-range goal is to pedal twenty miles per hour for a half hour. If you're older than fifty, your goal is to attain a speed of twenty miles per hour for at least twenty-three minutes. When you finish your exercise, release the tension control and pedal without any resistance until your heart rate returns to normal.

Now back to our eager ex-smoker who has just run two traffic lights, nearly bowled over somebody's grandmother, and is furiously pedaling against traffic in a frantic attempt to burn off some calories. Whoa, buddy, slow down! Concentrate on a nice smooth rhythm. Don't push so hard. Don't strain at the pedals because it overexerts the legs and can cause muscle cramps. You'll end up wanting to take a nap instead of finishing your day's workout.

If you plan to bicycle outdoors, wear a helmet. Even professional racers often take spills and it's important to protect your head. Use a light and reflectors on the wheels if you plan to bicycle at night. Purchase a pair of shoes with cleats. Also, curtail your exercise program—or make it a real quick one—when outdoor air pollution levels are high. And when

Bicycling Distance in Minutes and Days to Lose Five Pounds

(Calculated at approximately 7 mph) Example: If you reduce your calories 400 per day, and bicycle thirty minutes for twenty-five days, you will lose five pounds. If you reduce your caloric daily intake by 1,500, it will take thirty minutes of bicycling for nine days to lose five pounds.

Minutes	Days	Amount of Calories Reduced Per Day
30	25	400
45	22	400
60	19	400
30	17	800
45	14	800
60	13	800
30	9	1,500
45	8	1,500
60	7	1,500

you're purchasing a bicycle, buy it from a reputable sporting goods store. Take it for a test ride as you would a car.

Like walking, bicycling affords you the leisurely opportunity of meeting people and seeing something of your neighborhood as well. Not only is it an enjoyable form of exercise, but it beats subway crowds and expensive bus fares. Many cities provide special bicycle routes so that people can pedal their way to and from work. If your city or town provides such lanes, take advantage of them.

Bicycling uses up about 6.5 calories per minute depending on the terrain, type of bike, and your own speed, skill, and ability not to get hit by a car. If you bicycled a leisurely seven miles per hour, you would burn up approximately 390 calories in one hour. Increase that speed to 12 miles per hour and you would lose 410 calories.

Walking

Walking, like bicycling, is better than a singles' bar if you want to meet people and get some fresh air at the same time. Best of all, on a brisk walk you also use up about 5.2 calories per minute. The exact amount of calories you expend will, of course, vary according to your weight, the terrain, and the duration of the walk.

How does the amount of caloric expenditure vary with weight? Well, when it comes to exercise, the heavier you are the more calories you use up doing a particular exercise. An average man who weighs 154 pounds uses 5.2 calories per minute by walking. If you weighed more than this, your caloric burnoff would be higher. Conversely, it would be lower if you weighed less. Based on our "average" man's weight, in order to achieve our goal of a 300-calorie burnoff per exercise session you would have to walk fifty-nine minutes—almost an hour—and that makes walking an ideal lunch-hour activity.

Walking is not only beneficial for weight loss, but as you will later learn it's also an ideal way to combat any stressful feelings you may have as a result of giving up cigarettes. If you're feeling depressed, moody—even angry—go out and take a walk. Breathe deeply as you do so.

Let's take our new exercise program one step at a time. When it comes to this activity, distance is your goal—not speed. A half hour of brisk walking will do you as much good as running fast for twenty minutes, but it must be done on a regular basis. During such a brisk walk your heart rate increases to 70 percent of its maximum level, which is an ideal rate both for aerobic benefit and calorie burnoff.

Walking fits so easily into the most hectic personal and professional schedules that it is the ideal form of exercise. You don't need any special equipment or training, and a regular program of walking is the perfect exercise to build up your cardiovascular strength should you want to switch to a more demanding form of exercise such as jogging or swimming.

For us ex-smokers, walking is such an effective physical activity in our battle against weight gain that it's possible to lose as much as twenty-five pounds in little more than two months by cutting down on calories and taking a brisk thirty-to-sixty-minute walk each day.

There are a few simple pointers you should be aware of when pounding the pavement. Posture is important, so when you walk stand tall—don't slouch. Pull in that gut and try to tighten up your buttocks. Keep your head high and spine straight. When you walk, swing your arms and develop a bouncy step. All this will help you get off on the right foot.

It might start to sound redundant, but it's not a bad idea to do a few warm-up exercises before you go for your daily stroll. The following suggested exercises concentrate on stretching muscles in the lower back area, and will help contribute to the prevention of lower back problems:

STANDING REACH AND BEND—Stand erect with your feet shoulder-width apart. Extend your arms over your head. Stretch as high as possible while keeping your heels on the ground. Hold this position for fifteen to thirty seconds. Repeat a second time.

FLEXED-LEG BACK STRETCH—Stand erect with your feet shoulder-width apart. Keep your arms at your side. Slowly bend over, touching the ground between your feet. Keep your knees flexed. Hold this position for fifteen to thirty counts. If at first you can't reach the ground, touch the top of your shoe line. Repeat a second time.

ALTERNATE KNEE PULL—Lie on your back, feet extended and hands at your side. Pull one leg to your chest, grasp it with both arms, and hold for a five count. Repeat with opposite leg. Repeat this exercise seven to ten times with each leg.

DOUBLE KNEE PULL—Lie on your back, feet extended and hands at your side. Pull both legs to your chest, lock arms around legs, and pull buttocks slightly off the ground. Hold this position for twenty to forty counts. Repeat seven to ten times.

TORSO TWIST—Lie on your back, knees bent, feet on the ground or secured under something to prevent them from lifting during this exercise. Lace your fingers behind your neck. Curl your torso to an upright position and twist, touching the right knee with the opposite elbow. Return to your starting position. Repeat twisting in the opposite direction. Exhale on the way up, inhale on the way down. Repeat five to fifteen series.

While there are many ways to begin your walking program, we thought we might offer an example of one that is highly recommended by fitness experts. If such a program doesn't fit your needs, you may alter it. Also, if you find a particular week's pattern tiring, repeat it before going on to the next pattern. You do not have to complete this program in twelve weeks.

Week 1: Walk slowly five minutes. Walk briskly five minutes. Walk slowly five minutes. Total time, fifteen minutes. Do this a minimum of three times a week.

Week 2: Walk slowly five minutes. Walk briskly seven minutes. Walk slowly five minutes. Total time, seventeen minutes. Do this a minimum of three times a week.

Week 3: Walk slowly five minutes. Walk briskly nine minutes. Walk slowly five minutes. Total time, nineteen minutes. Do this a minimum of three times a week.

Week 4: Walk slowly five minutes. Walk briskly eleven minutes. Walk slowly five minutes. Total time, twenty-one minutes. Do this a minimum of three times a week.

Week 5: Walk slowly five minutes. Walk briskly thirteen minutes. Walk slowly five minutes. Total time, twenty-three minutes. Do this a minimum of three times a week.

Week 6: Walk slowly five minutes. Walk briskly fifteen minutes. Walk slowly five minutes. Total time, twenty-five minutes. Do this a minimum of three times a week.

Week 7: Walk slowly five minutes. Walk briskly eighteen minutes. Walk slowly five minutes. Total time, twenty-eight minutes. Do this a minimum of three times a week.

Week 8:   Walk slowly five minutes. Walk briskly twenty minutes. Walk slowly five minutes. Total time, thirty minutes. Do this a minimum of three times a week.

Week 9:   Walk slowly five minutes. Walk briskly twenty-three minutes. Walk slowly five minutes. Total time, thirty-three minutes. Do this a minimum of three times a week.

Week 10:   Walk slowly five minutes. Walk briskly twenty-six minutes. Walk slowly five minutes. Total time, thirty-six minutes. Do this a minimum of three times a week.

Week 11:   Walk slowly five minutes. Walk briskly twenty-eight minutes. Walk slowly five minutes. Total time, thirty-eight minutes. Do this a minimum of three times a week.

Week 12:   Walk slowly five minutes. Walk briskly thirty minutes. Walk slowly five minutes. Total time, forty minutes. Do this a minimum of three times a week.

Check your pulse periodically to see if you are exercising within your maximum target zone, As you get into shape, try to exercise within the upper range (75 percent) of your heart-rate zone. Remember, your goal is not only total fitness and weight loss, but enjoying your activity as well.

As we said earlier, walking is a great exercise because it's a practical approach to weight loss. Also, there is no need to purchase any expensive equipment. You can wear your everyday clothes anytime or anyplace you may decide to undertake your walking program.

If, however, the weather turns cold, it's a good idea to wear clothing that keeps you warm but isn't too heavy. Lightweight ski jackets are excellent for walking. Remember to keep your extremities covered in cold weather. Tennis socks are also a good idea in low temperatures.

If you are engaged in a walking program during hot weather, light slacks and a sportshirt or T-shirt are recom-

Calories Expended in Walking

Weight	Miles Per Hour	Distance	Calories
90	3	2.4 miles	100
90	3	4.8 miles	200
90	3	7.1 miles	300
90	3	9.5 miles	400
110	3	2.1 miles	100
110	3	4.1 miles	200
110	3	6.2 miles	300
110	3	8.3 miles	400
130	3	1.8 miles	100
130	3	3.6 miles	200
130	3	5.5 miles	300
130	3	7.3 miles	400
150	3	1.6 miles	100
150	3	3.3 miles	200
150	3	4.9 miles	300
150	3	6.5 miles	400
170	3	1.5 miles	100
170	3	2.9 miles	200
170	3	4.4 miles	300
170	3	5.8 miles	400
190	3	1.3 miles	100
190	3	2.7 miles	200
190	3	4.0 miles	300
190	3	5.3 miles	400
210	3	1.2 miles	100
210	3	2.5 miles	200
210	3	3.7 miles	300
210	3	4.9 miles	400
230	3	1.1 miles	100
230	3	2.3 miles	200
230	3	3.4 miles	300
230	3	4.5 miles	400
250	3	1.1 miles	100
250	3	2.2 miles	200
250	3	3.2 miles	300
250	3	4.3 miles	400

mended gear. Try to walk in the shade; a pair of sunglasses will help keep you comfortable. A hat is in order whether the weather is hot or cold. If it's really a sizzler, there's nothing wrong with turning on your air conditioning and taking a few turns around the house.

One inexpensive piece of equipment you might want to invest in is a pedometer. It's easy to carry when you're walking and a pedometer will tell you exactly how far you've walked. If you plan to follow the walking program described here, it is important that you wear a watch.

Not all shoes are made for walking. If the shoe fits, wear it. A shoe which fits properly should be a half inch longer than your foot. There must be room up front for toe movement. A soft, supple upper made of leather or fabric is best. Jogging or running shoes are excellent, but so are basketball sneakers provided they have an arch for support and have a broad rounded toe. The shoe must have a good grip on the back of your foot to keep your heel from sliding or rubbing.

You now know everything you wanted to know but were afraid to ask about walking. Now let's see how many calories will be consumed on that next jaunt around the block. Find your own weight in the left-hand column and you'll see how far you have to walk to lose from 100 to 400 calories. You'll note on the chart on page 88 that a lighter person burns fewer calories; a heavier person burns more for the same amount of activity.

Jogging

Jogging, like rock and roll, seems here to stay. It's become the choice of the Pepsi Generation, and big city marathons have become media events which attract runners from all over the world. Keep in mind that jogging may be too strenuous an activity for the long-dormant ex-smoker. In fact, if you are over forty and haven't been active, you should begin with a walking program instead. After completing the walking program outlined in this chapter, you can begin with Week 3 of the jogging program we will outline a bit later in this section.

What we're going to do right here is give you a "walk test" to determine which of the three following programs you should follow now that you've decided to run. We will start by finding out how many minutes—up to ten—you can walk at a brisk pace, without undue difficulty or discomfort, on a level surface.

If you cannot walk for five minutes without experiencing discomfort, kick off your jogging regimen with the first week of Program A. If you can walk more than five minutes, but less than ten, you should begin with the third week of Program A.

If you can walk for the full ten minutes, but are somewhat tired and sore as a result, you should start with Program B, which combines walking and jogging. If you can breeze through the full ten minutes, you are ready for bigger things. Wait until the next day and take the "walk-jog test." In this test you alternately walk fifty steps (left foot strikes the ground twenty-five times) and jog fifty steps, for a total of ten minutes. Before taking the test, read the jogging guidelines which appear a bit later on.

If you cannot complete the ten-minute test, begin at the third week of Program B. If you can complete the ten-minute test, but are tired and winded as a result, start with the last week of Program B before proceeding to Program C, which is the most advanced. If you can perform this test with no difficulty at all, begin with Program C.

A word of caution. If during any of these tests you experience nausea, trembling, extreme breathlessness, pounding in the head, or pain in the chest, stop immediately. If the symptoms persist beyond the point of temporary discomfort, check with your physician.

All right, before we begin let's do some of the stretch and reach exercises outlined in the section on bicycling. It's vital to warm up before any exercise. We'll add a few more exercises here that are especially geared to jogging enthusiasts.

ACHILLES TENDON AND CALF STRETCHER— Stand facing a wall approximately three feet away. Lean forward and place the palms of your hands flat against the wall. Keep your back straight, your heels firmly on the ground. Slowly bend elbows to hands. Tuck your hips toward the wall. Hold this position for thirty seconds and repeat the exercise with your knees slightly flexed.

HURDLER'S STRETCH— Sit on the floor with one leg extended straight ahead. The upper part of the other leg should be at a right angle to your body, with the heel close to the buttocks. Slowly slide hands down extended leg and touch foot. Hold this position for thirty seconds. Keeping legs in same position, slowly lean back and rest elbows on the floor. Hold this position for thirty seconds. Reverse positions and repeat both stages of the exercise.

BACK STRETCHER— Lie on your back with your legs straight and arms at sides with palms down. Slowly lift your legs, hips, and lower part of your back and attempt to touch your toes to the floor behind your head. Keep your legs straight and hold this position for thirty seconds.

THIGH STRETCHER— Stand at arm's length from the wall with your left side toward the wall. Place your left hand on the wall for support. Grasp your right ankle with your right hand

91

and pull your foot back and up until your heel touches your buttocks. Lean forward from the waist as you lift. Hold this position for thirty seconds. Repeat the exercise with your opposite hand and foot.

STRADDLE STRETCH— Sit on the floor and spread your straight legs to about twice your shoulder width. Slowly lean forward from the waist, sliding your hands along the floor as far forward as you can. Hold this position for thirty seconds. Return to your starting position. Slowly stretch forward over your right leg, sliding both hands down to the right ankle. Try to keep your knee straight and touch your chin to your right kneecap. Hold this position for thirty seconds. Return to your starting position and repeat the second step of this exercise on the left side.

LEG STRETCHER— Sit in same position as in preceding exercise. Rest your left hand on your left thigh and grasp the inside of your right foot with your right hand. Keep your back straight and slowly straighten your right leg, letting it rise to about a 45-degree angle. Hold this position for thirty seconds. Repeat this exercise with the other leg.

All stretched out? Feeling nice and limber? All right, let's outline the three walking/jogging programs. Program A is for those former smokers who showed the least stamina during the "walk test."

Program A: Walking Program

Week 1:   Walk at a brisk pace for five minutes, or for a shorter time if you become uncomfortably tired. Walk slowly or rest for three minutes. Again walk briskly for five minutes, or until you become uncomfortably tired.

Week 2: Same as the first week, but increase pace as soon as you can walk five minutes without soreness or fatigue.

Week 3: Walk at a brisk pace for eight minutes, or for a shorter time if you begin to feel uncomfortably tired. Walk slowly or rest for three minutes. Again walk briskly for eight minutes, or until you become uncomfortably tired.

Week 4: Same as the third week, but increase pace as soon as you can walk eight minutes without soreness or fatigue. When you have completed Week 4 of this program, begin Week 1 of Program B.

Program B: Walking/Jogging Program

Week 1: Walk at a brisk pace for ten minutes, or for a shorter time if you become uncomfortably tired. Walk slowly or rest for three minutes. Again walk briskly for ten minutes, or until you become uncomfortably tired.

Week 2: Walk at a brisk pace for fifteen minutes, or for a shorter time if you become uncomfortably tired. Walk slowly for three minutes.

Week 3: Jog twenty seconds (50 yards). Walk one minute (100 yards). Repeat twelve times.

Week 4: Jog twenty seconds (50 yards). Walk one minute (100 yards). Repeat twelve times. When you have completed Week 4 of this program, begin Week 1 of Program C.

Program C: Jogging Program (Consult jogging guidelines which follow.)

Week 1: Jog forty seconds (100 yards). Walk one minute (100 yards). Repeat nine times.

Week 2: Jog one minute (150 yards). Walk one minute (100 yards). Repeat eight times.

Week 3: Jog two minutes (300 yards). Walk one minute (100 yards). Repeat six times.

Week 4: Jog four minutes (600 yards). Walk one minute (100 yards). Repeat four times.

Week 5: Jog six minutes (900 yards). Walk one minute (100 yards). Repeat three times.

Week 6: Jog eight minutes (1,200 yards). Walk two minutes (200 yards). Repeat two times.

Week 7: Jog ten minutes (1,500 yards). Walk two minutes (200 yards). Repeat two times.

Week 8: Jog twelve minutes (1,700 yards). Walk two minutes (200 yards). Repeat two times.

You are now getting increasingly stronger as a jogger, just as you are becoming increasingly fitter as an ex-smoker. So keep up the good work. Jogging, by the way, is an excellent means to help keep you smokeless. That's because it's quite difficult to enjoy this activity if you do smoke and, secondly, your improved physical condition encourages a desire within you to improve other aspects of your life.

Jogging Guidelines

You don't need any expensive lessons or equipment to learn how to jog, but here are a few basic guidelines that will help you to excel at your new exercise program:

1. Run in an upright position. Avoid the tendency to lean. Keep your back as straight as you can and still remain comfortable. Keep your head up. Don't look at your feet.

2. Hold your arms slightly away from your body, with the elbows bent so that the forearms are approximately parallel to the ground. By occasionally shaking and relaxing your arms and shoulders, you will reduce the tightness that sometimes develops while you are jogging. Periodically taking several deep breaths and blowing them out completely also will help you to relax.

3. It is best to land on the heel of the foot and rock forward so that you drive off the ball of the foot for your next step. If this proves difficult, try a more flat-footed style. Running only on the balls of the feet, as in sprinting, will produce severe leg soreness.

4. Keep your steps short, letting the foot strike the ground beneath the knee instead of reaching to the front. Length of stride should vary with your rate of speed.

5. Breathe deeply, with mouth open. Do not hold your breath.

6. If for any reason you become unusually tired or uncomfortable, slow down, walk, or stop.

Once you begin jogging regularly, your long-range goal should be to run for one hour at 75 percent of your maximum heart-rate level. A short-range goal should be jogging a distance of two miles at an eight-to-ten-minute pace. You can work up to three miles, five times a week at the same pace if you feel up to it.

Another nice thing about jogging is that it's an inexpensive activity. You don't have to pay to do it, and the only special equipment you will need is a good pair of running shoes. Shoes with heavy, cushioned soles and arch supports are recommended over flimsy sneakers or racing flats. Your running shoes should be a half size too large when you try them on: your feet will swell when you run.

Weather will dictate the rest of your attire if you jog outdoors. A good rule of thumb is to wear lighter clothing than temperatures might seem to indicate, because you'll be working up a good sweat. Light-colored clothing that reflects the sun's rays is cooler in the summer, and dark clothes are warmer in the winter. When the weather is very cold, it's better to wear several layers of light clothing than one or two heavy

Calories Expended in Jogging

Weight	Distance, miles	Calories
90	2.1	100
90	4.2	200
90	6.3	300
110	1.7	100
110	3.4	200
110	5.1	300
130	1.5	100
130	2.9	200
130	4.4	300
150	1.3	100
150	2.5	200
150	3.8	300
170	1.1	100
170	2.2	200
170	3.3	300
190	1.0	100
190	2.0	200
190	3.0	300
210	0.9	100
210	1.8	200
210	2.7	300
230	0.8	100
230	1.6	200
230	2.5	300
250	0.8	100
250	1.5	200
250	2.3	300

layers. The extra layers help trap heat, and it's easy to shed one of them if you become too warm.

You should wear some kind of head covering when you are running outdoors during the winter or summer months, and you shouldn't wear any garments which interfere with the evaporation of perspiration. On extremely hot and humid days it's best to run in the morning or evening.

Remember to do stretching exercises before and after your run no matter how far or how long you decide to jog. Also remember to cool down when you finish any physical activity. Listen to your body when you run. If you develop pain or any other unusual symptom, slow down or stop. If the problem persists, go see your doctor. And don't compete with others until you are an experienced, well-conditioned runner. Your objective is to prevent or do something about weight gain and to steadily improve your own performance—not to run faster than someone else. Unlike smoking, jogging is a "positive addiction," so get hooked.

The table on page 96 shows how many calories you use up while jogging at the leisurely pace of six miles per hour. Just find the weight closest to your own and you'll see how far you would have to jog to burn off 100, 200, or 300 calories.

Swimming

Swimming made a splash way back in history, just as it is popular today among health-conscious people throughout the world. During the years when Persia was a superpower, men drafted for military training were required to take swimming lessons. The ancient Greeks, meanwhile, both male and female, participated in a variety of swimming activities, because the Greeks believed that the ability to swim was as important as reading and writing.

In this country, swimming is rated by many exercise specialists as the best way to keep in shape or get into top physical condition. Swimming is also recognized as America's most popular active sport. Private health clubs—including most YMCAs—offer convenient noon and dinner-hour lap swims. Interestingly, the amount of calories one expends while swimming does not vary with weight, but with skill. In fact, the less skilled you are at this sport the better! If you can barely dog paddle your way across a pool, take heart! You're using up more calories in your plodding efforts than the speedsters. Swimming washes away about 8.5 calories a minute, so to use up 300 calories plan to splash about for thirty-five minutes.

We're not going to teach you how to swim in this section, but we are going to show you some water exercises you can do whether or not you know how to swim—exercises that will help you work off any unwanted pounds. But first a few words for all you ex-smokers out there who do know how to make it from one end of the pool to the other.

Lap swimming is an excellent weight-loss activity. But you don't have to keep up a nonstop routine of only swimming laps in order to shed pounds. Kick off the side of the pool and swim hard until you begin to feel winded. Ease off by loafing with a lazy breaststroke or sidestroke until you catch your breath. Once you feel recovered, then swim hard again. About a half hour of this type of activity is recommended. The basic idea is simply to stay in motion.

If you haven't done any regular swimming for some time, slowly wade into this activity. Swimming, by the way, is highly recommended for anyone over sixty who has just quit smoking and is looking for a good form of exercise. What you should do is set a goal for yourself of 100 yards. After about five minutes of swimming, remember to stop and check your heart rate to make certain you are in the safe target range. If you're more than fifty years old, set a 50-yard goal for yourself when first starting out. Try to swim a minimum of three times a week, and add another 50 yards to your workout every two weeks. Your long-range goal is to swim about 600 yards in fifteen minutes.

Another good way to kick off your exercise program in the pool is to swim one length of the pool, get out, walk back, and repeat this routine several times. It's also a great way to catch the attention of that good-looking lifeguard! Gradually increase the number of lengths you swim before walking back, until you are swimming five or ten lengths before walking back to your starting point.

As with any other activity, it's important to warm up before doing any exercising in the pool. The stretching and bending exercises described in the section on bicycling are also perfect for this type of activity. Most swimming activities cause the back to be excessively extended, so do these exercises before and after you complete a workout.

If you don't know how to swim, the best aerobic exercise you can do is to stand waist-high in the water and jog in place. You simply stand with your arms bent in a running position and pretend you're on a running track. Read the jogging section to determine how long you should keep at this exercise.

Another good aerobic exercise for the nonswimmer is the standing crawl. Simulate the overhand crawl by reaching out with the left hand, getting a grip on the water, pressing downward and pulling, bringing the left hand through to the thigh. Reach out with the right hand and repeat this exercise.

Bouncing is also a good weight-loss exercise that can be done while standing in chest-deep water. Bounce on your left foot while pushing down vigorously with both hands. This will cause the upper body to rise. Repeat this exercise with the right foot.

You can also bounce in place with alternate arms stretching

forward. Stand in waist-deep water. You bounce in place with a high knee action. Your right arm is outstretched far forward when your left knee is high, and the left arm and hand are stretched rearward. When the right knee is high, the left arm and hand are stretched forward, with the right arm and hand stretched rearward. When changing arm and knee positions, pull down and through with your hand simulating the propulsion of the crawl stroke.

Water-treading exercises are excellent for swimmers. You can do no-hand treading, one-hand-held-high treading or two-hands-held-high treading exercises. Other water exercises include pedaling in water, in which you start from a back-lying position in the water. You simulate a pedaling motion with knees raised alternately to the chest, using reverse sculling to stay in the same place in the pool.

These and many other exercises are described in detail and with diagrams in a publication issued by the President's Council on Physical Fitness and Sports. The publication is produced in cooperation with the National Spa and Pool Institute.

Remember to have fun in the water. You can play water tag, throw a "party" with some friends at the bottom of the pool, do backward and forward tumblesaults, or even bring your snorkel equipment. Water activities will help improve your flexibility, coordination, strength, and, if sustained for twenty or more minutes, will improve your aerobic condition and help you lose weight.

Equipment is minimal. In a chlorinated pool it's advisable to wear a pair of goggles. If you don't like water in your ears or up your nose, ear and nose plugs are also recommended.

The table shows how many miles you would have to swim to work off some of these calories. We're clocking the swimmer in this chart at about two miles an hour. Just find your own approximate weight in the left-hand column, and read across.

Calories Expended in Swimming

Weight	Miles	Calories
90	1.9	100
90	3.7	200
90	5.6	300
110	1.5	100
110	3.0	200
110	4.5	300
130	1.3	100
130	2.7	200
130	4.0	300
150	1.2	100
150	2.3	200
150	3.5	300
170	1.0	100
170	1.9	200
170	2.9	300
190	0.9	100
190	1.8	200
190	2.7	300
210	0.8	100
210	1.6	200
210	2.4	300
230	0.7	100
230	1.4	200
230	2.1	300
250	0.7	100
250	1.3	200
250	2.0	300

Calories and Exercise

All right, we've spent a considerable amount of time extolling the virtues of exercise. What does it all really mean to the former smoker? Let's take, for example, a popular food item

Minutes of Exercise
(based on average weight of 154 lbs.)

Food or Beverage	Calories	Walking	Bicycling	Swimming	Jogging
Beer (8 oz.)	115	22	18	14	12
Wine, Burgundy (4 oz.)	110	21	16	13	11
Coca-Cola (8 oz.)	105	20	16	12	11
Bread (fresh toasted white, rye, whole wheat, Italian, or French, 1 slice)	60	12	9	7	6
Biscuit (2-inch diam.), with honey (1 tsp.)	164	32	25	19	16
Pancake with butter (1 pat) and syrup (2 tbsp.)	240	46	36	28	24
Chocolate fudge (1¼-inch sq.)	118	23	18	14	12
Popcorn (1 cup), butter (1 tsp.) and salt	295	57	44	35	30
Spaghetti and meat sauce, Italian (1 serving)	295	57	44	35	30
Oreo cookie (1)	40	8	6	5	4
Butter (1 pat)	35	7	5	4	4

Food					
Cottage cheese (1 rounded tbsp.)	30	6	4	4	3
Ice cream (½ qt. or 5 rounded tbsp.)	186	36	28	22	19
Milk (2% fat, 8 oz.)	126	24	19	15	13
Yogurt (from skim milk, 1 cup)	122	24	18	14	12
Cheesecake (1 slice or $\frac{1}{12}$ of a 9-inch cake)	160	30	25	19	16
Egg, fried or scrambled with oil (1 tsp.)	108	21	16	13	11
Apple, raw (2½-inch diam.)	87	17	13	10	9
Avocado, raw (½)	167	32	25	20	17
Orange, raw (3-inch diam.)	73	14	11	9	7
Lemonade (8 oz.)	105	20	16	13	11
Hamburger, cooked (3-inch diam. × 1 inch thick)	224	43	34	27	22
Bacon, fried (2 strips)	90	17	14	11	9
Hot dog, 1 frank, 8/lb. package	170	32	26	20	17
Lamb chops, 2 (3 oz. ea. cooked)	205	39	31	25	21
Peanuts, roasted (6–8 nuts)	86	17	13	10	9
Chicken leg, fried (1 med.)	282	54	42	34	28
Shrimp, deep-fried (3½ oz.)	225	43	34	27	23
TV dinner, chicken, fried	542	104	81	65	54

Minutes of Exercise (Concluded)

Food or Beverage	Calories	Walking	Bicycling	Swimming	Jogging
Sausage pizza (⅛ of 14-inch pie)	195	38	29	23	20
Lettuce, iceberg (⅛ of 4¾-inch head)	10	2	2	1	1
Potato (1 med.), baked, with sour cream (2 tbsp.)	140	27	21	17	14
Tomato, raw (3-inch diam.)	40	8	6	5	4
Mushrooms, fresh, raw (10 small or 4 large)	28	5	4	3	3
Corn, sweet (1 ear)	70	14	10	8	7
Broccoli (1 5½-inch stalk)	32	6	5	4	3
Oysters, raw (5–8 med.)	66	13	10	8	7
Corned beef sandwich	240	46	37	29	24
Blue cheese salad dressing (1 tbsp.)	70	14	10	8	7

Adapted from EXERCISE EQUIVALENTS OF FOODS: A PRACTICAL GUIDE FOR THE OVER-WEIGHT, by Frank Konishi. Copyright © 1973 by Southern Illinois University. Reprinted by permission.

such as a baked potato. A baked potato with sour cream weighs in at a hefty 140 calories. In order to peel those calories away, you would have to walk twenty-seven minutes, bicycle twenty-one minutes, swim for seventeen minutes, or jog for fourteen minutes. That's part of what exercise is all about.

We've included a chart listing some popular foodstuffs so that you can see at a glance how your favorite dish rates in terms of energy expenditure. Now that you're on an exercise program, and although you know you can work some or most of these calories off, this chart may help you decide whether or not you really want that slice of cheesecake . . .

How long would you have to walk, bicycle, swim, or jog to work off the calories from those tempting pancakes you couldn't resist for breakfast? Anywhere from twenty-four minutes to forty-six minutes, depending on what form of exercise you may choose.

S · I · X

EVEN EX-SMOKERS
GET THE BLUES

By now we hope you've jotted down in the chart we've provided for you in Chapter 1 some of the mood swings you may be experiencing. Have you been yelling at your cat more often than you should? Were you a little testy on the phone yesterday while talking to your mother? Did you wake up this morning and want to go right back to sleep?

These types of feelings—stress, anger, depression, boredom, etc.—are, as we've already mentioned, some of the emotional aftershocks that rock even the most mild-mannered new ex-smoker. Unfortunately, many former smokers who do not understand what is happening to them race off to a therapist's office—a needless waste of time and money. That is why it is important for you to understand that such mood swings are a natural progression of the smoking withdrawal process and can be dealt with on your own.

Let's take a look at a mood which will probably be on most lists—depression.

* * *

Perhaps one of the most personally devastating—and least known—side effects of giving up smoking is depression. Once the initial euphoria of being an ex-smoker subsides, you may begin to feel like a miserable version of your old self. Such blue funks can lead to many negative things—an eating binge is just one of them. What is causing such feelings? Once again, the villain in the piece may be that incredibly powerful drug, nicotine.

The latest research on the subject indicates that depression may be caused by the lack of a substance we all have in our bodies called norepinephrine. This substance belongs to a chemical grouping called, simply enough, amines. Norepinephrine, along with other amines, is contained in a minuscule sac in every one of some 10 billion nerve cells in the brain.

The purpose of these amines is to assist in the transmission of electrochemical impulses from one nerve cell in the brain to another. We can compare these individual nerve cells in the brain to shortwave radios, broadcasting and receiving messages. If a nerve cell is turned on, or transmitting messages, these amines close the gap between two nerve cells and prepare the next cell for signal reception. They form a sort of bridge— a synapse, in scientific terminology—so the two cells can communicate. If that bridge is somehow blocked or destroyed by other chemical compounds, that nerve cell, for the moment, is not transmitting. It is turned off.

The amount of norepinephrine in each nerve cell is delicately balanced. If this balance is tipped toward a deficiency and the cells are locked in an "off" position, some scientists believe this norepinephrine deficiency can lead to depression. On the other hand, a surplus of norepinephrine can produce just the opposite effect. Scientists now know that hallucinogens such as LSD and other drugs like amphetamines produce dramatic increases of norepinephrine levels. The drug user is literally "turned on." His nerve cells are transmitting constantly because their "switch" is locked in an "on" position.

An exciting, ground-breaking study now also links smoking to increased norepinephrine levels in the brain. This remarkable piece of research was conducted at Washington University's School of Medicine. Ten men ranging in age from twenty-four to forty-two were selected for the study. All were smokers. Within a ten-minute period five men smoked two cigarettes, while five subjects sucked drinking straws to simulate smoking. During the course of the experiment, blood levels of norepinephrine were measured at regular intervals for thirty minutes.

The straw smokers showed no changes in their norepinephrine levels, but the norepinephrine levels of smokers rose to a peak of 45 percent above normal fifteen minutes after they puffed their first cigarette. After twenty minutes, the norepinephrine level fell to about that of the nonsmokers.

It seems likely from the available evidence that the "lift" smokers get after lighting up a cigarette is not a psychological one, but a *physical* one. It is a "high" that any of us who ever smoked may actually have become addicted to. And when we quit smoking, with our blood level of norepinephrine no longer raised periodically by the effects of nicotine, we can go into an emotional tailspin.

Norepinephrine isn't the only nicotine-stimulated substance that can affect our moods. Nicotine also raises blood levels of chemicals called endorphins. But, whoa! Let's back up a bit and get some background on these unique substances called endorphins.

Endorphins are often referred to as the "body's own opiates." Their presence wasn't even discovered until recently when they were found by a team of researchers at Stanford

University. The researchers were trying to determine how morphine, heroin, and other opiates work in the brain to produce a high. What they found is that the effects of opiates are unleashed by the attachment of the drug molecule to a part of tissue called a "receptor"—a chemically designed surface on certain nerve cells in the body uniquely adapted to fit opiates.

The fact that these "receptors" are so uniquely adapted to fit opiates led the scientists to ask the breakthrough question: Why would nature provide these surfaces when the only known opiates in natural form are from the opium poppy—and relatively few of us ever encounter these? The scientists believed the answer must be that the body somehow manufactured its own opiate substances to fit these receptors. The endorphins (literally meaning "morphine within") are those opiate substances.

The first endorphins researchers discovered were a rather weak breed. It wasn't until 1976 that the potent morphinelike substances called beta-endorphins were identified by scientists.

Like opiates derived from the poppy, endorphins cause changes in the body that can both relieve pain and profoundly affect our mood. In fact, scientists found that endorphins so dramatically affect mood that the symptoms of both depression and schizophrenia (split personality) can be temporarily alleviated by the injection of beta-endorphins into the bloodstream.

Dr. Nathan S. Kline, who pioneered this astonishing research with his patients at the Rockland Research Institute in New York State, observed that his patients underwent several distinct stages of improvement after such an injection.

Just minutes after the injection patients reported that their depression had lifted. Several said they felt elated, as if they had taken a stimulant drug. This reaction lasted two to three hours followed by a period of drowsiness. The last and most dramatic reaction tended to occur about twelve hours later, and remained in effect from one to ten days. During this period

Kline observed that symptoms of depression or schizophrenia either lessened or actually disappeared. Some patients even exhibited personality traits that had been buried for years due to their illnesses.

Because the effect of nicotine in raising norepinephrine and endorphin levels is so important to us new ex-smokers, as you shall shortly see, it is important to first take a look at another ground-breaking study which also dramatized the role of nicotine in causing such chemical reactions.

This study, conducted by the noted researcher Dr. Ovid Pomerleau, involved eight male smokers ranging in age from twenty-three to fifty-nine. The subjects varied in the number of years they had smoked. The twenty-three-year-old subject, for example, had smoked for only five years, while a fifty-five-year-old participant had smoked for forty-five years. The number of cigarettes smoked per day ranged from half a pack to three packs per day for the fifty-nine-year-old smoker.

During the experiments the subjects relaxed in an easy chair and listened to soothing music. A console in front of them dispensed cigarettes which were standard low- and high-nicotine cigarettes provided by the Tobacco and Health Research Institute at the University of Kentucky. The low-nicotine cigarette supplied 0.48 milligrams of nicotine, which is comparable to the low-tar-and-nicotine brands commonly sold everywhere. The high-nicotine cigarette weighed in at a hefty 2.87 milligrams—much higher than any brand found on the market.

One experiment took place on two consecutive days. On the first day the men were asked to smoke two low-nicotine cigarettes five minutes apart. The next day they were requested to smoke two of the high-nicotine cigarettes—also five minutes apart. After each session, blood samples were taken. From those blood samples the amount of nicotine and endorphins present was measured.

What Pomerleau and his fellow researchers discovered was that, after the subjects smoked the low-nicotine cigarettes, the amount of nicotine in the blood remained low and so did the level of endorphins. However, after they smoked the high-nicotine cigarettes, the amount of beta-endorphins in the blood had nearly doubled! Here was clear evidence that nicotine increases endorphin levels as well as norepinephrine levels.

So why is all this information so important? Because it challenges long-held beliefs about quitting smoking.

One commonly held belief is that people have such a difficult time giving up the cigarette habit because they can't handle the withdrawal symptoms. This notion holds that to ward off such effects, the smoker resumes the habit. But both these studies show that this is a misconception! Why we continue to smoke, in great part, is because nicotine is positively rewarding us by releasing both norepinephrine and beta-endorphins—those pleasure-producing substances.

This is extremely important for all ex-smokers to know. Why? Because as you will see in the next chapter, that "high" which is now missing in your life and may have you thinking about lighting up again can be recaptured through healthier outlets than tobacco smoke . . .

S · E · V · E · N

HOW DO YOU SPELL RELIEF?

Until now words like norepinephrine and beta-endorphins were not exactly part of your vocabulary, nor on your mind. But right now, as you endure some of the withdrawal symptoms we've been discussing, you're probably ready to climb the Empire State Building if that's what it takes to get hold of some of those funny-sounding compounds.

Well, there's a much easier way to again experience those calmer seas. Astonishingly enough, recent research shows that aerobic exercise—one of America's favorite pastimes—also raises blood levels of endorphins. To understand how this is possible, let's take a close look at a recent important exercise study.

This research project utilized seven female volunteers between the ages of eighteen and thirty. None of the women were involved in any regular athletic training program.

The rigorous two-month project consisted of a combination of conditioning exercises, bicycle ergometer rides, and running

113

for a total of one hour a day for six days a week. The women trained at 85 percent of their maximum heart rate during high-intensity activity (for a review of maximum heart rates, see Chapter 5). Within the one hour of daily exercise, the high-intensity activity was gradually increased from twenty minutes in the first week to thirty, forty, and finally forty-five minutes after three weeks, and then was maintained at the forty-five-minute level for the final four weeks of the program.

Monitored exercise "test" sessions were conducted before the beginning of the two-month program, in the middle, and immediately after its conclusion. In these test sessions, increases in the percentage of endorphin levels in the bloodstream were measured at intervals from zero to sixty minutes. There was a 57-percent increase of endorphin levels measured in the very first test session. The midpoint session saw a rise of endorphin levels to 79 percent, and the third test, conducted at the conclusion of the project, registered a whopping 145 percent increase in such levels. The results demonstrated that not only does exercise cause a rise of endorphin levels in the blood, but training enhances the effect.

Let's examine another study which utilized experienced runners to test endorphin levels. Six long-distance runners—five male and one female—were involved in the project. The test sessions consisted of thirty-minute runs, and blood samples were taken before and after each run period.

What blood analysis revealed is that levels of beta-endorphins had increased in the runners' bodies as much as two to five times after each session!

You might now ask why endorphins are released into the bloodstream during exercise. Scientists have several theories to explain this phenomenon. One theory speculates that endorphins regulate our perception of fatigue during exercise. We've probably all experienced that rather strange phenomenon of getting a "second wind" during exercise or some other strenuous activity. Some scientists believe that endorphins may be responsible for this sensation.

Another hypothesis is that a large increase of endorphins during exercise may be due to this compound's ability to control pain. During exercise, several pain-producing chemicals are building up in the blood. Such a buildup should result in pain—especially in trained athletes—but for some reason it does not. Quite the opposite happens, in fact. After a certain amount of physical exertion, runners, for example, experience that well-publicized sensation called "runners' high"—a euphoric state that is in part responsible for the positive addiction so many people have to this sport. To some scientists, it sounds like the doings of our good friends, the endorphins.

So, finally, what does all this scientific research mean to us new and almost new ex-smokers? It suggests that a good exercise program, in addition to preventing us from gaining unwanted pounds, can help beat the woes of nicotine withdrawal. It also means that the time to start such an exercise program is not tomorrow or next week, but right now!

Let's move on to another mood that's probably made our list of emotions—boredom. How often have you jotted down boredom next to any one particular activity—your job, for example? That was exactly the case with a friend of ours who first quit smoking and then decided to quit her job.

One day Gail explained to us that she smoked pretty heavily while working as a secretary in a university public-relations office. Gail said she never really understood why until the day she decided to give up cigarettes. It was at that moment, she explained, that she realized how much she depended on those "smoke breaks" to ease the monotony of her job.

Confronted with the choice of further endangering her health by smoking again or dumping her "boring" job, she made the wiser choice and quit. In our friend's case, these were only the first steps in a series of positive changes she was to make in her life. By the way, two years later Gail has not only found a better job, but she is still smokeless!

Maybe you're beginning to discover similar things about your own lifestyle. If after you've seriously committed yourself to breaking the cigarette habit you're now wrestling with the problem of boredom, perhaps there is the temptation to pick up a piece of candy in lieu of a cigarette.

But short of quitting your job or devouring an entire box of candy, what can you do about this problem? Part of the solution may lie in learning to *anticipate* the problem. Let's take an everyday situation as an example:

You've taken your car into the garage for an oil change. One alternative to impatiently hanging around the garage, and perhaps wishing for a cigarette so that the time would pass faster, is to use that time more productively by running some errands. Another option is always to carry something of interest to you—a new best-seller, a crossword puzzle, or even a tape deck. The point is to try creatively to avoid such boring situations.

Now, if you've jotted down boredom a lot, and not just in a few specific situations, maybe you should start thinking about creating some new goals or restructuring some old ones. Let's talk first about some short-term goals—goals, say, that you think you can achieve in about a year.

For example, you could go after that real-estate license you've always wanted or take that pottery or music appreciation course. Why not do some volunteer work? Start to attend cultural events. Participate in a hobby club—photography, gardening, stamp-collecting, or dancing organization. Join a support group, if necessary, or begin one of your own (more on the importance of support groups later). The opportunities are only limited by your imagination.

Like our friend Gail, maybe you too should start thinking in terms of some long-range goals that you've always wanted to achieve. Giving up cigarettes should give you the confidence to know you can accomplish such goals. For example, think about making a career change, starting your own business, or getting that graduate or undergraduate degree. Once again, your opportunities are only limited by your imagination, so get going!

Now let's discuss another emotion which may be appearing a bit too frequently on our list of moods—anger. Some research has indicated that nicotine has a modifying effect on this emotion, which is why, now that you no longer smoke, you may be experiencing more flareups than usual. One of the most effective ways we've discovered of deep-sixing anger is through deep-breathing exercises.

Breathing Exercises

You may doubt that breathing has any relation to our emotions, but there you're wrong. Our breathing patterns and emotions are very closely related. In fact, our breathing patterns change as our emotions change. Thus, we can alter our moods by breaking old breathing habits. A good example is an emotion we've just talked about quite a bit—depression. The next time you find yourself in a blue funk, try this simple experiment:

Stop whatever you're doing for a moment and analyze your breathing rhythm. Chances are you're probably not breathing very deeply, because most people who feel depressed take short, shallow breaths. And if you're really feeling bummed out, don't be surprised to find yourself sighing. Researchers say that sighing is frequently a sign of deep depression.

Now try the following deep-breathing exercise and watch your mood begin to lift. This exercise can be done while sitting, standing, or lying down.

1. With your mouth closed and shoulders relaxed, inhale as slowly and deeply as you can while silently counting to eight. As you are doing this, push your stomach out.
2. Hold that breath to the count of four.
3. Exhale slowly, again to the count of eight.
4. Repeat this inhale/exhale cycle five times.

What you're really doing in this exercise is shifting your source of breathing from the chest to the diaphragm. Shallow breathing, or thoracic breathing, is a signal of a stressful situation. Diaphragmatic breathing—from the stomach—is the road to relaxation.

Diaphragmatic breathing is the method most natural to man. We all breathe that way as infants. The next time you watch a baby breathe, you'll notice that there is little or no movement of the chest. What you will see is the stomach moving, which indicates diaphragmatic breathing.

When that same child is under emotional stress and begins to cry, the chest starts to heave rapidly in and out. The infant is now chest-breathing. Unfortunately, as we grow older, most of us form the lazy habit of chest breathing. Why? For a variety of physical, psychological, and cultural reasons.

Poor posture is one physical reason for breathing with the chest. When we slouch or slump, diaphragmatic movement is prevented, and we are forced to rely on thoracic breathing. Culturally, women are taught from an early age that it is more feminine to "keep your stomach in." But by not allowing the stomach muscles to extend outward, the stomach and liver are prevented from moving out of the way so that the diaphragm can flatten out. This literally forces women to breathe with their chests.

One key way we can begin to control the stress which affects the ex-smoker and people who have never smoked as well, is to gain better mastery over our breathing habits. We must all consciously begin to start breathing more deeply with our diaphragms rather than with our chests. Here is one exercise designed to do exactly that:

First, put your right hand on the top part of your stomach. Position your hand so that the little finger is located directly above your navel. Spread your fingers in such a way that your thumb almost touches your chest. Now, take your left hand and put it on your upper chest. Make certain that your little finger is between your two breasts. As you breathe, concentrate on your stomach alternately filling and emptying with air. Your right hand should be rising and falling, but your left hand should not move.

Proper breathing also serves another function. It will help to get rid of years of accumulated stale air and smoke that have been trapped within your lungs. According to researchers, this old air can actually lead to a desire to smoke because it prevents you from breathing fully!

That's why it's so important for ex-smokers to learn how to breathe properly. Once you relearn what has always come naturally to you, your body will be pumped with fresh oxygen which will not only help energize you, but also restore your natural skin color. Proper breathing will also help restore the elasticity which your lungs lost as a result of smoking.

All right, you've put out your last cigarette. Now try to take a really deep breath. Not so easy to do, is it? This is just one of many examples of the harm smoking can cause the human body. But don't worry about it; once you work on the following breathing exercises you'll be breathing as deeply as a long-distance runner. But you must do these exercises just as diligently as your physical workout program.

These breathing exercises are designed to satisfy your cigarette cravings and to replace the relaxing sensations you thought you got from smoking. Do them as often as you can.

In fact, anytime you feel like reaching for a cigarette or are experiencing stress or anxiety, select one or a combination of these exercises to do. Repeat the particular exercise four or five times—or more—if you feel the need to do so. When you complete an exercise or a series of exercises you should feel relaxed and energized.

We've talked some about ex-smokers' willpower in this book. Let's talk about it a bit more. If you wanted to reach for a cigarette and, instead, completed one of these exercises and did not smoke, take some time to reflect on your victory. You continue to make great strides in remaining smoke-free. This might be the perfect time to reward yourself in a manner of your own choosing.

Feeling stressful and tense is difficult for anyone—smoker and nonsmoker alike. During such moments you may feel like you're under the gun. So say you couldn't resist taking a puff of a cigarette. Don't despair. Don't discard everything you've worked for since quitting. Continue these breathing exercises along with your physical exercise program. Simply view what happened as a small setback and try again. (More on recidivism later.)

The following exercises, developed by Philip Smith, author of *Total Breathing,* make reference to "total breath." When instructed to take a total breath, it means you should fill your lungs to the maximum and put into play your chest, rib and stomach muscles. In other words, use every respiratory muscle and every inch of lung to their fullest.

No-Smoking Breath

This is a perfect exercise for use during the day, at the office, after dinner or whenever there is a tension buildup in the chest area that needs to be relieved.

1. Forcefully inhale the total breath. Breathe in as deeply as possible.

2. Hold the breath for two seconds.

3. Tilt your head slightly back and exhale through your mouth with great force. As you exhale, shape your lips into a tiny "O" so that the air has to be forced out during the exhalation. Pull in your stomach with the exhalation so that the air is really forced out.

4. After repeating this breath three or four times, finish off with a regular total breath.

5. After the initial cigarette craving has left, you may want to repeat this exercise, only a bit more gently. Often people find themselves yawning briefly after this exercise, as the body accommodates itself to a new supply of fresh oxygen.

Relaxation Breath

Although this exercise is somewhat similar to the previous one, the release of the breath relieves different areas of stress.

1. Gently inhale the total breath.

2. Hold the breath for three seconds.

3. Clench your teeth and open your lips. Force the air out between the teeth. You will be making a hissing sound like a teakettle.

4. Repeat four times. You may wish to vary the intensity of the exhalation and the hissing. For some people, a slight, almost inaudible hiss is more effective than a loud forceful hiss.

5. Return to normal breathing with the total breath.

"Ahh" Breath

Also good for relieving stress.

1. Gently inhale the total breath. Breathe in as deeply as possible. Fill the lungs, the chest, and then the midsection.

2. Hold the breath for three seconds.

3. Open your mouth and, as you exhale the breath, release a giant sigh, making a tension-releasing "ahhh" sound. Again, remember to exhale beginning with the abdomen and gently working upward until you have released all the air.

4. Return to normal breathing with the total breath.

Repeat this exercise if necessary. You may mix the two exercises. After three repetitions of the No-Smoking Breath, you may finish your relaxation exercise with the "Ahh" Breath.

Release Breath

The purpose of this exercise is to lower anxiety levels and reinforce the effect of proper breathing. It requires a bit of mental visualization as well.

1. Close your eyes as you inhale the total breath. Imagine that you are inhaling pure relaxation. You may want to use a visual image to reinforce this concept. Imagine a soothing color such as a cool blue or picture a perfect day at the beach and breathe in that clean, slightly salty, crisp air.

2. Hold for three seconds. During this period mentally gather up all the tensions in your body. Check your face, the muscles in your cheeks, around your eyes, and especially the back of your neck and your shoulders. Scan the rest of your body for any other tensions. Get ready to breathe

them out in the exhalation. Gather any remaining tension and dissolve it into the air that you now retain in your lungs.

3. Exhale through slightly rounded lips, as if you were going to whistle. As you exhale, actually feel those tensions leaving your body in a steady stream of air.

4. Inhale a complete deep total breath and exhale forcefully through an open mouth.

Lung Cleaning

The following set of breathing exercises is designed to extract larger and larger portions of stale dead air while increasingly ventilating the lungs. Ideally, these exercises should be performed at least twice a day, in the morning before work and in the evening before dinner. You might wish to add an additional set about an hour before bedtime, because sleep is the time during which the lungs and the skin rid themselves of accumulated toxins.

1. For this exercise you may stand or sit, but far superior results are achieved when you are standing.

2. Very slowly inhale the total breath. As you inhale, lightly pound your chest with the fingertips of both hands, moving them randomly about to cover the upper chest, breast area, and the sides of the rib cage. If you find yourself coughing, decrease the force with which you pound.

3. Hold the breath for five seconds and gently slap the entire area of your chest with flat open hands.

4. Exhale through rounded lips.

5. Inhale the total breath.

6. Retain for five seconds.

7. Now gently rub or caress your chest, upper chest, breast area, and the sides of your rib cage with flat open palms.

8. Exhale through rounded lips.

9. Inhale the total breath.

10. Retain for five seconds.

11. Exhale through rounded lips.

This exercise will stimulate both the muscles and the cells of the respiratory system. The light pounding or percussion will begin to ease and break up the congestion that prevents you from breathing more deeply. When you finish this exercise, your entire chest area will tingle and your breathing will be freer and easier.

Retained Breath

This exercise strengthens and helps increase the elasticity of the respiratory muscles, and also stretches out the lungs and the chest. By forcefully exhaling two times you remove residual air that prevents the body from being properly oxygenated.

1. Stand erect.

2. Inhale the total breath.

3. Hold the breath as long as possible. (This does not mean holding your breath until you are dizzy and about to pass out.) Start by holding this breath for about twenty seconds, then gradually work your way upward, adding another five or ten seconds whenever you feel comfortable in doing so.

4. Exhale forcefully through your mouth. As you finish the exhalation, pull your stomach in again and you will find that there is a second exhalation. Squeeze this last bit of air out of your lungs. In this way you will be continually cleaning out the reserve air that accumulates with each inhalation.

5. Return to total breathing. Repeat the entire exercise three times.

Piston Breath

The following exercise furthers the elimination of stale, useless air from the lungs.

1. Sit comfortably erect in a chair or on the floor.
2. Inhale the total breath.
3. Quickly exhale the breath through the nose by contracting the stomach as far in as possible.
4. As you release the stomach, simultaneously take in another total breath.
5. Repeat this inhalation and forceful exhalation ten times in a row. Your stomach should be rapidly moving in and out like a piston, and your breath should sound like a choo-choo train gradually picking up speed.
6. After ten times, inhale the total breath. Hold for five seconds and exhale.

Watching the Breath

This is another good exercise for relieving stress, and one designed to create a tranquil state. A bit later in this chapter you will be reading about the effects of yoga and meditation on stress, and the following is an excellent prelude to a meditation or yoga exercise.

1. Exhale completely.
2. Lower your eyes so that they focus intently on the tip of your nose. Your eyes may become a little "crossed" as you do. There is no danger.
3. Very slowly and gently begin to inhale. You should feel the breath entering at the tip of the nose. This sensation

should continue straight up the nose and into the top of the forehead. Even though you feel the stomach inflating and the ribs expanding, keep your attention focused just at the entranceway to the nostrils.

4. When you complete the inhalation, hold the breath for ten counts, which should be based on the pulse beat you feel just under your eyes or in your forehead.

5. Let the exhalation just quietly stream out the end of the nostrils. At the end of each exhalation you may wish to close your eyes for just a moment and let the waves of calmness wash through your entire head.

6. Then begin the next inhalation.

This exercise should be done while sitting in a comfortable chair with your hands in your lap. Repeat it three times at first, and later you may want to work your way slowly up to ten repetitions. This should come only after a month of practice.

Calming Breath

This exercise is also excellent for creating a calming sensation throughout the body when you are feeling *severely* stressful. As above, sit comfortably and try to relax.

1. With your right hand outstretched, fold down the second and third fingers into your palm so that your thumb, ring finger, and little finger remain standing.

2. Close your eyes. Place your right thumb against the right nostril, pressing it closed. Slowly begin to inhale the total breath. As you begin to inhale through the left nostril, direct the air in a smooth stream straight up to your forehead. Close your eyes and imagine that you are breathing in not just plain air but a very special air that is tinted with calming

colors. This may be white, blue, clear, or yellow. As the inhalation fills your body, let the color fill the body as well, bringing relaxation, strength, and harmony to all parts of the body.

3. At the end of the inhalation, clamp the left nostril shut with the fourth and fifth fingers of the right hand. Hold the breath and the colored air for ten counts. During this time imagine the air gathering up all the tensions and anxiety from the body and the one thousand and one unnecessary thoughts from the mind and consolidating them so that they may be expelled all at once with exhalation.

4. Now, keeping the left nostril closed, release the thumb that is holding the right nostril.

5. The color of the exhalation will be dirtier than that of the inhalation. This exhalation will carry out all the tensions and toxins that the inhalation has accumulated. For example, if you inhaled a calming light blue breath, the exhalation will be a muddy dark blue breath.

6. Repeat the entire breath, only this time reverse the procedure by clamping the left nostril with your fourth and fifth fingers and inhaling through the right nostril. The exhalation will be through the left nostril, with the right nostril held shut by the thumb. Again, you will inhale your preferred color breath, hold, and exhale. Repeat the entire breath four or five times or until the exhalation is the same color as the inhalation.

Breathing Tips

Now that you're beginning to employ breathing techniques that will help you through those stressful moments, here are some handy tips that will assist in maximizing the success of your breathing program:

While you should take full advantage of the breathing exercises we've just described anytime or anywhere you might feel the urge to smoke, it is best to practice these techniques early in the morning. Always try to find a quiet place in your home for the duration of the exercise, even if it means disconnecting your telephone for a while. Keep the room temperature comfortable and wear loose clothes.

If an exercise calls for you to be seated, it's best to sit cross-legged on something soft—a rug, pillow, blanket, etc. If this position causes you any discomfort, sit with your back and pelvis against a wall. Kneeling and sitting on your feet is also a good way to do your breathing exercises.

Before we move on, here is one final breathing exercise that you may find useful. While this exercise suggests that you use a straw, you might look a little silly sitting at your desk and sucking on a straw. A cigarette holder will do just as well and it's not as obvious.

The exercise was developed by Carola Speads, who has been involved in teaching proper breathing since she was seventeen, and is the author of a book on the subject, *Breathing: The ABC's*. When doing this exercise, try to avoid gulping air and holding it in before you start. Also avoid forcing air out at the end of your exhalation. Gentle inhalation and exhalation are the idea.

This exercise is not only good for those moments when you're thinking about a cigarette, but is also helpful should you have a sudden craving for a snack.* It should take between

---

* Another technique Speads suggests for when that craving for a smoke gets to you involves the use of a carrot. It is a technique, she says, that has worked for hundreds of ex-smokers.

Carry raw carrots with you immediately after you've put out your last cigarette, she advises. And when that sudden urge to smoke strikes, start chewing on one. Carrots, Speads explains, are so tough to chew on—it takes so much time to eat one—that by the time you have finished chewing up your raw carrot the urge to smoke will have passed.

three and five minutes for this exercise to help stem your appetite.

1. Put a straw or cigarette holder in your mouth and let the air pass through it instead of your nose.
2. Try not to help the flow at all—don't force the air through the straw.
3. Raise the straw up to your mouth instead of bending down to it. This will prevent pressure or strain on the neck and chest.
4. Inhale gently.
5. Take the straw out of your mouth shortly before the end of your exhalation and let the rest of the air pass through your nose.

Yoga

As we have now learned, proper breathing can be beneficial in the relief of stressful feelings. Blue funks, depression, and other negative emotions can be helped by certain breathing techniques.

Several Eastern traditions have long stressed the importance of breathing regulation in achieving emotional self-control. In this country Yoga is the most popular of these traditions.

Yoga is a Sanskrit word which translates into "reunion"— a harmony of body and mind. There are a variety of yogas, and some of the teachings and practices date back at least 5,000 years. Yoga is not a religion, so whether you be Catholic, Protestant, or Jew it will not offend any of the tenets of your faith. Instead, yoga is a system of philosophy developed in ancient India.

There are, according to yogic tradition, several "paths"

or "ways" to peace, harmony, and the glorification of the supreme being. Bhakti yoga, for example, stresses love and devotion as a way to attain communion with God, while Hatha yoga—the most popular form of yoga to be practiced in the Western world—emphasizes breath, posture, and movement. A third yoga, Raja yoga, teaches meditation and self-realization. You may read more about any of these systems in books to be found at your local library or bookstore, but for now we're going to concern ourselves only with Hatha yoga.

Hatha yoga is an exercise system that is designed to expand the conscious awareness of both the mind and body. Its ultimate purpose is to lead its followers systematically from physical exercises to breathing exercises to mental exercises—all of which are supposed to lead one to a higher state of consciousness.

We would guess, however, that as an ex-smoker you are at this point less interested in higher consciousness than in ways to reduce some of the stress you may be feeling. It is this same concern which is drawing the interest of growing numbers of researchers who deal with stress.

An increasing number of behaviorists, for example, are currently using techniques steeped in Hatha yoga. They are using fancy terminology—like "Stress Inoculation Training" or "Anxiety Management"—but the roots of these systems are Hatha yoga.

There are even several schools of psychotherapy which maintain that there is a "crucial link" between breathing patterns and emotional functioning—something suggested by the yogic masters thousands of years ago. Followers of the late Wilhelm Reich suggest that "respiration is related to the flow of feeling and where that flow is inhibited by muscular tension the feelings are blocked." In a similar vein, practitioners of the Gestalt school of psychotherapy view the inability to breathe correctly as "correlated with the experience of anxiety."

Again, none of these revelations are new. These principles were being utilized not only by the yogic masters, but by adherents of Zen Buddhism and Sufism as well.

There are many beneficial yoga exercises, but here is one that will help calm the ex-smoker who is feeling tense, anxious or outright jittery.

1. Sit upright on something comfortable.

2. Close your eyes (if riding a bus, train, or other public conveyance, you can keep your eyes open—especially if you're trying this on a subway in New York).

3. Forcefully exhale all the air out of your lungs.

4. Inhale through your nose to a slow count of eight. Do it like this: First fill your stomach to a four count. Then fill your chest with air as you count to seven. On the eight count fill your shoulder blade area with air.

5. Now exhale to the same eight count—go slowly. Count to two and empty the shoulder blade area. Now, count three to five and empty the chest area. With the remaining three counts, empty your stomach of air.

6. Do this two more times.

7. Stop, relax, take it easy for a few minutes.

You have now done the basic yoga relaxation technique. Your mood should be measurably improved and you may even be feeling a burst of energy. That's because Hatha yoga produces not only a profound relaxing effect, but an energizing one as well.

Hypnosis

Hypnosis is rarely given its due as an effective tool in inducing a relaxation response in people suffering from stress or anxiety.

Despite its long history of clinical usage, most people still associate hypnosis with the hocus-pocus of the carnival midway.

But, in fact, the hypnotic state can best be described as that of complete relaxation, both physical and mental. Like yoga, hypnosis also has its roots in antiquity. The ancient Greeks practiced it as a form of therapy for anxiety and hysterical states. The mystical Druids called it "magic" sleep and used it to cure warts and to cast spells.

Modern studies using sophisticated electronic equipment to examine brain rhythm patterns suggest that a hypnotized person is neither awake nor asleep, but somewhere between these two states. It seems that hypnosis induces what is called a "relaxation response," one which is characterized by a decrease in heart rate, respiration, and blood pressure. This response, according to researchers, is the opposite of the "fight or flight" response in which the body reacts to emergencies. In such an emergency situation heart rate, blood pressure, and respiratory rate all increase.

Even though the hypnotic state is brought about by the voice of the hypnotist, the actual hypnotic state is something that the subject really accomplishes by himself. In fact, most people are hypnotized several times a day without even realizing it. When you have driven forty miles and can't remember the last thirty, you were probably in a mild hypnotic state. Daydreaming is a mild form of self-hypnosis.

Because many people still have a variety of misconceptions about hypnosis—and because such misconceptions might prevent you from giving it a try—let's answer a few of the most commonly asked questions.

Q. Who can be hypnotized?

A. Studies indicate that only about 10 percent of people are unable to be hypnotized. Which means almost anyone is capable of being hypnotized.

Q. What makes a good subject?

A. Mainly the ability to let go and cooperate. Poor hypnotic subjects are those who keep evaluating what the hypnotist is saying, or find the situation ridiculous.

Q. Can I be made to do something I don't want to do?

A. No. Contrary to popular literature, a person is never a slave to a hypnotist. You are aware of all suggestions and will simply refuse to do anything against your wishes.

Q. Is hypnosis dangerous?

A. No more dangerous than sleep.

What is important to us ex-smokers is that we make use of all the tools we have available to us in our battle against nicotine addiction, stress, or any other negative emotions. Hypnotism is one such tool, and many smokers have reported success in giving up cigarettes through the use of hypnosis. It may also be used successfully in keeping you smoke-free.

You owe it to yourself at least to investigate the possibility, whether or not it works for you. In the meantime, there are many informative books on the subject at your local bookstore or library, so read up on the subject.

Meditation

Meditation, like hypnosis and yoga, is another relaxation technique with its roots in antiquity. A person who meditates turns his total attention and awareness upon a single object, concept, sound, or experience. In this country and throughout most of the Western world, the goal of meditation is not to attain religious ecstasy, but to reduce stress, eliminate anxiety, and induce increased feelings of relaxation.

It is apparent that meditation works in the same way as

hypnosis in inducing a relaxation response. Thus, blood pressure, heart and respiratory rates, and even oxygen consumption seem to decrease during a meditative state.

Several years ago, New York City's telephone company decided to investigate the effects of meditation on the mental health of its employees. Workers volunteered for a six-month study and practiced a simple form of meditation. When the study ended, those employees who participated in the experiment reported that they felt more able to cope with the stresses of daily life. Volunteers also said that meditation helped them overcome moments of depression and even reduced feelings of hostility.

There are many schools of meditation, and a variety of methods exist to attain a meditative state. People who have been meditating for years like to spend an hour each morning at this mental exercise. If you are just beginning to meditate, your short-term goal should be approximately ten minutes. Gradually work your sessions up to a half hour. An excellent, nondenominational prayer to precede your morning meditation has been written by the Brothers of the Abbey of the Genesee in Piffard, New York. It is to be recited as follows:

> *This is the beginning of a new day. The Lord has given me this day to use as I will. I can waste it, or I can use it for good. What I do today is important because I am exchanging a day of my life for it. When tomorrow comes, this day will be gone forever, leaving in its place something I have traded for it. I want it to be gain, not loss; good, not evil; success, not failure; in order that I shall not regret the price I paid for it.*

The following is a simple meditation technique that can be used each morning or anytime stress, depression, or a case of the blues gets you to thinking about a cigarette. Your goal is to clear your mind of all negative thoughts and open yourself to the soothing balm of the meditational process.

1. Sit quietly in a comfortable position and close your eyes. Find a room where you won't be disturbed.

2. Close your eyes and deeply relax your body. Relax all the muscles. Begin at your feet and work up to your face. Keep them relaxed.

3. Breathe through your nose. Become aware of your breathing. Concentrate on it. As you breathe out, say the word *one* silently to yourself. For example, breathe in . . . out, *one;* in . . . out, *one;* etc. Do this from ten to twenty minutes. You can open your eyes to check the time, but do not use an alarm.

4. While you are doing this, other thoughts or images may float through your mind. Don't fight them, try to ignore them. Keep counting your breaths. If there are any distracting noises, ignore them as you would those errant thoughts.

5. When you finish sit quietly for several minutes at first with closed eyes and later with open eyes.

6. Don't worry about whether you were successful in achieving a deep level of relaxation. This is relaxation practice. Enjoy it and don't try too hard.

Deep Massage

Massage is an ancient healing art that is highly effective for relaxing those muscles tense due to stress. In fact, the Chinese and Japanese 3,000 years before the Christian era were already practicing various massage techniques.

If you are feeling muscular tension—tightness around the neck or in the back muscles—you may want to investigate this technique in order to rid yourself of such tension. Massage not only relaxes muscles, but helps generally to tone the entire body as well.

Many new ex-smokers also complain of fatigue. When you are tense, or under stress, your muscles are expending extra energy as they tighten up. This may be one reason why you are feeling fatigued, experiencing headaches, or generally feeling stiff all over. Massage may be the remedy. It's also excellent for those days when you may be feeling nervous or a bit irritable as a result of going smokeless.

There are many massage techniques. All are geared to the same end—to break down muscular tension and prevent it from returning. But you should choose a system that is more than the sensual rub-down that you read about in many magazines.

One of the best of these techniques is the deep massage. Unlike the more superficial rub-downs which only manipulate the muscle surface, deep massage can reach structures far below the surface of the body. It is considered the most potent technique for releasing long-standing tension and pain.

Deep massage involves stroking, kneading, and applying strong pressure to the muscles. But if you find that this technique is a bit too much for you, choose a different system. It is important to be in the hands of a masseur or masseuse who is skilled in a variety of techniques and who will select one best suited to your needs.

Pins and Needles

A rather new addition in this country to the list of healing arts is an ancient and distinctly Chinese one—acupuncture. It may turn out to be one of the most effective weapons yet in the arsenal of tools to deal with the effects of nicotine withdrawal.

American interest in acupuncture actually began to develop after President Nixon's visit to China in 1972. Since then, many physicians have returned from journeys to China marveling at major operations they witnessed where the only anesthetic used was acupuncture.

Today, acupuncture is being applied to other uses in this country. It is being used to treat chronic pain, deafness, and, most recently, has been studied as a treatment for narcotic withdrawal—and yes, even nicotine withdrawal. Let's take a took at one acupuncture treatment program and its success in helping 194 people quit smoking.

The subjects, who varied in age from fourteen to sixty-seven, were given three acupuncture treatments to help them break the smoking habit. All the volunteers abstained from smoking the Monday morning prior to their first session. As a result, many people showed up already in the first throes of cold turkey.

Despite this condition, the volunteers reported feeling so calm and relaxed after the acupuncture session was completed, that the desire to smoke had actually vanished. According to the study, these positive effects lasted until the next treatment the following day. Since the symptoms of nicotine withdrawal had lessened somewhat by the second treatment, this session provided even longer relief, and the subjects did not have to return until Thursday for their third and final treatment.

After completion of all three treatments, 95 percent of those participating in the study had quit smoking. Eighty-five percent of those treated reported that acupuncture was successful in easing the aftereffects of nicotine withdrawal. Now, that's quite a recommendation!

Unfortunately, after two years only 30 percent of those original participants remained smokeless, which is about the success rate of other "quit smoking" programs. Then why bother to use acupuncture? Because what is clear from this study is that acupuncture can definitely help us weather those annoying withdrawal symptoms in the first critical week or so of not smoking. And to some that may mean the difference between licking the habit or returning to it.

Let's back up a bit and take a look at what acupuncture is and how it works.

According to Chinese folklore, it all started thousands of years ago when a soldier, pierced by an arrow, felt sudden relief from a chronic pain in a part of his body that was nowhere near his wound.

Out of this remarkable discovery—or so the story goes— the Chinese evolved a system of medicine that cured by penetrating the skin at certain points. That system was founded upon the belief that our body has the inherent ability to heal itself. We can see examples of this in our everyday life. For example, when we get dust in our eye, tears naturally form to wash it away. Similarly, a scraped hand heals with little effort on our part. It is believed that acupuncture simply stimulates the natural healing powers within the body.

The traditional Chinese theory of how acupuncture is believed to heal and diminish pain lies in balancing the body's negative-energy (yin) and positive-energy (yang) life forces. According to Chinese thought, disease reflects an imbalance of these energy forces. The traditional acupuncture practitioner first attempts to identify the nature of the imbalance of energy and then selects the appropriate acupuncture points on the basis of that evaluation. There are about 1,000 such points in the body.

Once the relevant point is identified, a very slender needle or needles (varying from two to a dozen or more) are inserted and left there for any time from a few seconds to a few minutes. The needles used to be rotated by hand, but now many practitioners use electrically stimulated needles.

One theory of how acupuncture works is of particular interest to new ex-smokers. In this theory, we find the endorphins described earlier in this book playing a central role. It is hypothesized that acupuncture needles relieve pain by stimulating nerves in the muscles which, in turn, send messages back to the brain to release endorphins. These endorphins then block the transmission of pain messages.

The good news for us ex-smokers is that since both acupuncture and nicotine apparently cause the release of endorphins, we can use acupuncture like exercise during those first crucial weeks of giving up cigarettes—as a means of combating the effects of nicotine withdrawal!

Laugh and the World Laughs with You . . .

They say that laughter is the best medicine, and for us ex-smokers that's almost literally true. Have you ever tried to smoke or eat while you're laughing? Well, you can't. So laughter is one thing we recommend plenty of.

The philosopher Epictetus astutely observed centuries ago that "Men are disturbed not by things, but by the view they take of them." Humor is really a way of standing back a bit from taking things too seriously—putting a little distance between you and the problem at hand. By doing that, you're bound to get a different perspective on things.

In his autobiography, *Anatomy of an Illness,* writer Norman Cousins even credits humor, in part, for his recovery from a serious and very painful disease. He discovered that ten minutes of real belly laughter had much the same effect as an anesthetic. In fact, Cousins says that laughter brought him such relief from pain that he could sleep for two hours without any other medication.

Which leads us to—you guessed it—the subject of endor-phins again. According to one research study, laughter may stimulate the release of these helpful compounds. So don't sit there feeling blue, find something to laugh about . . .

E · I · G · H · T

YOU ARE WHAT
YOU EAT (I)

We've already seen that negative emotions such as depression and stress can be pretty powerful "triggers" in our smoking and eating habits. We've also established that positive emotions—such as feeling happy or relaxed—can also serve as triggers and lead to overeating or smoking.

By now you've probably filled out the chart we provided you with earlier in the book. Let's now take a look at it and note how often you've jotted down that you're in a relaxed state. Perhaps even at this moment you're parked in front of your video recorder with a tray of snacks instead of a pack of cigarettes. Having that tray of snacks handy is not a good idea. What we ex-smokers constantly have to be vigilant against is substituting food for cigarettes.

One possible alternative is to find a different means of relaxing—preferably something that involves use of your hands to keep you from nibbling food. Perhaps you could busy yourself planting an exotic indoor herb garden, or finish crocheting that sweater you started for your dog last year. You might even repair that door that never closes properly or try your hand at a crossword puzzle.

Another option involves a more direct assault on the problem. If you find yourself snacking, immediately remove all food from the recreation room so that it is not readily available when you have a desire to eat something.

As a second line of defense, store any high-calorie food items in the back of your refrigerator or cupboard so that they are not easy to get to. Shelve your low-calorie snacks in the front. Very often, preplanning a snack defuses the impulse to eat. Plan to save a portion of your last meal to use later as a snack. Since that snack is no longer "forbidden fruit," you may not even desire it any longer.

For the hopeless nibbler, excellent snacks for ex-smokers are fruits that must be peeled or nuts which must be cracked. These items keep both your hands and mouth busy. And according to one recent magazine article, there's even some evidence that eating alkaline-forming foods, such as fresh fruit, nuts, whole grains, or yogurt, can actually help reduce the craving for a cigarette.

Foods to avoid those first critical weeks after you've quit smoking are acidifying products, such as meat, sugar, alcohol, cheese, and eggs.

Now let's examine your eating patterns during the meal itself. As a smoker, you probably always hurried through a meal just for the reward of lighting up that cigarette. Now, as a former smoker, you still hurry through a meal but may be replacing that cigarette with a second helping of dessert.

The most effective way to attack this problem is to portion out your meals and immediately put away any leftovers. If that second helping of roast and potatoes is already cooling in the refrigerator, you're less likely to want it. A more drastic measure is to immediately dispose of any leftovers or spoil any food that tempts you too strongly. If the sight of food makes you hungry even if you aren't, then salt your desserts and sugar your potatoes.

Now is also the time to begin to work on modifying the habit you developed as a smoker of rushing through a meal. You must work on strategies aimed at slowing down the time it takes you to eat. Make a meal last at least twenty minutes. That shouldn't be too difficult because the food you're eating probably tastes better now that you've quit smoking. So enjoy it! Eating less and more slowly allows you to do exactly that.

Here are a few tips that will help you modify your old eating habits:

1. Cut your food into smaller bits.

2. Put your fork on your plate between mouthfuls. Chew your food thoroughly and swallow your food before picking up your fork again.

3. Sip water frequently during a meal. It will help you suppress your appetite.

4. Set a goal to be the last one finished at mealtime and, remember, no seconds!

We've now reached that part of the meal which is the most difficult for any ex-smoker to handle. As we said earlier, if there is one universal "trigger" which prompts smokers to light up, it's a meal's end. But now you must post a new stop sign—and it's not that slice of banana pie. To help you do so, we're going to serve up a few suggestions of our own:

1. Especially if you've just quit smoking, put social convention aside for a while. Get up from the table immediately after you've finished eating. Go brush your teeth. This will help remove the taste of food which tends to bring on the craving for a cigarette. It also adds a touch of sweetness, which will help you forgo that tempting piece of pie.

2. Serve coffee, brandy, or any other after-dinner beverage in another room to get away from the kitchen or dining-room table.

3. And if you simply must include dessert on the dinner menu, make it a low-calorie one such as fruit, plain cake, or a cookie. And if you must have a cup of coffee and you usually pour two teaspoons of sugar into your cup, now make it one.

These are small changes, but they represent a beginning—and an important one at that. Now let's continue your survival training at the dinner table or anywhere else where food is concerned . . .

YOU ARE WHAT
YOU EAT (II)

The previous chapter was a taste of things to come. You are not only going to have to think yourself thin, but eat yourself thin as well. Your normal eating habits and daily routines will have to change if you are going to survive as a nonsmoker. For example, some people eat when they're not even certain whether they're hungry. Others eat because they're stimulated by environmental cues such as the sight or smell of food or the arrival of the mealtime hour.

This is the type of behavior that must change. And we're going to try and help you do exactly that. To take that first step, remember to keep that detailed record of your eating habits which we spoke about earlier in this book. Keep such a record for at least a week. It might even be a good idea to carry this food record with you at all times. Write down what, when, where, why, and how you eat. Then review the record, asking yourself the following questions:

1. How many meals and snacks do I eat each day?
2. How much do I eat and how much time do I spend at each meal?
3. Is my eating behavior different on weekends than during the week?
4. Where do I do most of my eating?
5. Do I usually eat alone or with other people?
6. Do I eat only when I'm hungry, or also when I'm bored, nervous, stressful, or fatigued?

In reviewing your answers, you'll probably be astounded at some of the eating habits you've established without even realizing it. Such behavior is the key to the tale of the scales, so now let's tip those scales in your favor.

First of all, it's important that any changes you may now undertake as an ex-smoker—whether it be a new exercise program or a different approach to the dinner table—be done gradually so that you do not become discouraged.

For example, you may have better initial success changing the place where you usually eat rather than trying to control a tendency to eat when you're bored. This is an easy step to accomplish. If you usually sit in the living room and eat there as you read or watch television, that location—especially if the television set is on—may stimulate you to eat even if you aren't really hungry. You must become aware of this impulse— try to dissociate yourself from such a trigger—and make a decision to eat only when you're seated in the kitchen or some other specified area of your house.

Once you've accomplished such a change, reward yourself—buy something new, go to the movies, or take a leisurely walk in the park. This is a big first step. Meanwhile, continue to keep those records. Look them over for the good days as well as the not-so-good ones.

Now that you've begun to make changes and are trying to relearn old eating habits, here are a few suggestions that will help you on your way. It should take about a year for you to benefit from these tips.

1. Try eating one pat less of butter or margarine each day and watch 3½ pounds gradually melt away in a year.

2. Eliminate one slice of bread daily and you will lose six pounds within twelve months.

3. Guzzle one less beer each week and you will weigh 2½ pounds less in a year.

4. Eat ten potato chips less each week and by year's end watch yourself lose 1½ pounds.

5. You'll be 1½ pounds thinner a year from today if you say no to two slices of bacon each week.

6. You can lose up to four pounds in 365 days if you eat two doughnuts fewer each week.

7. And you can say bye-bye to five pounds in twelve months if you refuse one piece of cake each week.

You will discover other easy-to-follow tips throughout this chapter, and we do hope that you will follow them. What is most important, however, is that you fully understand what changes you need to make and why. You must strive for goals— step by little step—until you've developed a permanent set of appropriate eating habits which will help you win the battle of the bulge.

Here are a few more tips:

1. Just as preplanning a snack often defuses the impulse to eat, so it is with meals. Haphazard eating is often high-calorie eating.

2. Write your shopping list when you're not hungry. Go shopping on a full stomach. That way you won't be tempted

to buy extra goodies. It's a good idea to shop without your children around, because kids tend to load up grocery carts with all kinds of calorie-laden junk.

3. Eat only when seated at the kitchen or dining room table instead of nibbling while doing other things.

4. At mealtime, allow yourself only one moderate serving. Try portioning out your food before bringing it to the table.

5. Use smaller dinner plates or glasses to make your portions of food and beverage seem larger.

6. Remember to eat slowly. The goal is to extend each meal as long as possible because the brain's satiety center lags behind actual consumption.

7. Choose foods that you'll have to work at eating. For example, it takes longer to eat an orange than to drink a glass of orange juice. It also provides bulk and gives you something to do with your hands if you feel the urge to reach for a cigarette.

8. When you get the urge to eat between meals, do something else instead. Call a friend or walk the dog.

By now you've gotten a pretty good idea about ways to reduce your food intake. There are dozens of other suggestions you can follow, such as staying out of the kitchen unless you're the cook, or not licking the beaters or mixing spoons if you have to bake. And remember: no munching while watching television. As we said before, try to keep your hands busy— knit or sew, fold the laundry, organize your tool kit, groom your pet, or balance the checkbook. If all else fails, do some household chores in other rooms.

We've already discussed the value of exercise. Any increase in energy expenditure burns off calories. So why not make it a conscious decision to add some extra steps to your daily routine and really watch those pounds melt away?

We say conscious effort because, let's face it, we live in a sedentary world. All the miracles of modern technology—from electric can openers to power steering—have made life easier, more comfortable, and much less physically demanding. Americans, in fact, seem to pride themselves on time-saving devices that keep them from having to take an extra step.

So it's high time that you as an ex-smoker try out some new steps. We're asking you to put a bit more effort into your daily routines, and here are some suggestions about how to do exactly that:

1. When driving to work, park your car in the remotest corner of the parking lot—or park at least a half mile away from your destination—and briskly walk to and from your car.

2. Do the same thing when taking the bus or train. Get off a couple of stops early and briskly walk the remaining distance.

3. If you must run an errand that's not too far away, why bother with the bus, train, car, or cab? Walk instead.

4. In fact, why not run one superfluous errand each day on foot?

5. Take a stroll when you feel that early-afternoon nap coming on.

6. Climb stairs—don't ride elevators or escalators if you have a choice. This will burn off twice as many calories as walking on a level surface will. If you take the stairs two steps at a time, you'll burn off even more calories.

7. Take a vacation where activities include lots of walking.

8. Don't have your newspaper delivered. Instead, go out each morning and buy one.

9. When the telephone rings in your home, don't reach for the nearest extension. Go into the other room and answer it. Stand rather than sit while talking on the phone.

10. Replace coffee breaks with exercise breaks.

11. When your favorite television show breaks for a commercial, don't just sit there. Take a walk around your apartment.

12. Try doing some sit-ups while watching television.

13. Push the vacuum cleaner or lawn mower a little harder. Mop or sweep the floor more vigorously.

14. Avoid the drive-in window at the bank. Walk inside instead.

There are countless other ways in which you can increase your activity both at home and at the office, and you should take advantage of these opportunities. Take a positive attitude. Don't view such extra activity as an annoyance, but as an added boost to your weight-loss program. How effective are these little extra efforts? Here are some examples of calories used up in nonstrenuous thirty-minute activities:

Activity	Calories
Mowing	245
Sweeping	50
Ironing	38
Washing dishes	36
Carpentry	85
Standing	70
Gardening	110
Piano playing	30

You now have an idea of how important it is to modify your daily routine if you're concerned about those extra pounds. We will continue to talk about behavior modification in the next chapter because, as someone who has just quit or is about to give up smoking, you must make a commitment to change in many aspects of your life. Your old ways of doing and thinking about things when it comes to diet and exercise must be unlearned, because you're into a newer and healthier lifestyle now.

T · E · N

FOOD FOR THOUGHT

Changing long-established behavior patterns not only requires a willingness on your part to commit yourself to a new lifestyle, but will also require a little help from family and friends. In fact, in one weight-reduction program at the University of Pennsylvania's Day Hospital family members are encouraged to lend a helping hand.

The theory is that if people who care for you—be they family or friends—can learn more about what you're trying to accomplish, they can then help you reach your goals. So don't be shy about asking friends or family for moral support. Such support can help bolster your self-determination to remain smokeless and thin. Positive feedback can also help to reinforce your new eating habits.

In some cases you will have to deal with well-meaning friends or relatives who just won't understand what you're trying to accomplish. If, for example, someone tries to show affection for you with a gift of food, explain briefly that as an ex-smoker you're on a strict regimen to keep your weight down. If it's candy you're offered, try something like, "It looks wonderful, but don't tempt me. I'm sure you know somebody who isn't on a diet who would love to have these chocolates." If this doesn't work, put the gift aside quietly and give it away later.

Often people will change their own eating habits—refuse a piece of pie—in fear of tempting you. Tell them that they need not alter their eating patterns on your behalf. Don't discourage anyone from doing their own thing at the dinner table. You just do yours.

Enough about pitfalls. Now let's move on. Not only is it important to remain aware of the type and amount of food you eat; you must also pay attention to *how* the food you eat is cooked.

Try to eat only foods that are broiled, baked, steamed, or boiled—and with the fat trimmed away before cooking. You can enhance the flavor of foods you cook by adding herbs or dry wine. Learn to use herbs and spices instead of flavorings and sugar. Avoid deep-fried foods. Deep frying boosts the caloric content of any meal—and that includes vegetables.

However, if fry you must, use safflower oil. Use a skillet with a stick-free surface so that you don't have to cook with fats or oils. A good rule of thumb is to poach what you would ordinarily fry, and steam foods you would usually sauté. Load up on vegetables—they're great for you. Don't avoid potatoes. A medium-sized baked potato only contains about ninety calories.

If you usually eat out, monitoring how your food is cooked can be a bit more difficult. Your best bet is to eat at a vegetarian restaurant. Second choice is a Chinese restaurant because you can often have your meals cooked to order at such a restaurant. Seafood restaurants are also a good choice, but watch out for butter and tartar sauce. If you can manage it, order your seafood cooked plain—no butter, sauce, or gravy.

When you cook at home, aside from avoiding creams, butters, and sauces, don't use flour in the preparation of your meals. If you must have some kind of dressing on your salad, stay away from mayonnaise or oil dressings—too fattening. Instead, substitute vinegar, lemon juice, or a slice of lemon on salads and vegetables. You should also make use of sugar substitutes instead of the real thing. Also try to avoid alcohol because it is fattening.

Snacking is always a temptation—one that none of us can always overcome. If you must snack, pay as much attention to your reasons for snacking and to the kinds of treats you're eating as you pay to your regular meals. Here are some tips that may help you from going overboard when you snack.

1. Prepare your snack as you would a meal. Even if it's only a bag of chips, try eating the chips off a plate.

2. Log all your snack breaks in the record book you are keeping of your eating habits. Try to determine a pattern. Are there certain times that you reach for that bag of potato chips? If, for example, you discover that most of your snacking is done while watching that horror program on Saturday night, find something else to do that time of night.

3. Keep in mind that water helps to satisfy hunger pains. A diet cola, club soda, or natural fruit juice will also help satisfy that craving for a nosh. Avoid any beverage that has refined sugar in it. Remember, you can always sweeten a sugar-free beverage with peppermint extract, cinnamon, or even a twist of orange peel. Ice water served with a twist of lemon or lime is your best sugar-free drink.

4. Fresh or dried fruits are good snacks. Vegetables are the perfect snack. As we've said earlier in this book, one advan-

tage of eating fresh fruit is that it may need to be peeled; if not, washing it is probably in order. Such small operations help you avoid the tendency to eat too quickly, therefore decreasing caloric intake.

5. If a starchy snack is on your mind, remember that a baked potato contains comparatively fewer calories than other starchy foodstuffs. Cereals made with puffed wheat or rice are also low in calories.

6. Some good, low-calorie snack ideas include crunchy raw zucchini squash, broccoli, green peppers, celery, and carrots. You can also treat yourself to a tangy popsicle made by freezing six fluid ounces of fruit juice concentrate with eight ounces of plain, lowfat yogurt.

Remember, it may be easier to stick to your diet when you divide your daily calories into several meals and snacks—which means you don't have to skip your coffee break simply because you're on a diet. The key is to *plan* your meals and snacks. Choose foods that are low in calories but nutritious.

Many new ex-smokers, especially those concerned about weight gain, often rush out to the special low-calorie food sections of their local supermarkets. This is unnecessary. It's also costly. Diet foods are expensive and many are not much lower in calories than regular foods. Also, many experts believe that appetite-control drugs should be avoided. Such experts believe that these diet pills are only crutches and will not work for you in the long run.

Before you dash off to purchase a year's supply of appetite suppressants, give the weight-control techniques outlined in this book a chance to work. Above all, be patient. It should take about ten weeks to lose twenty pounds, and weight loss may vary depending on how active you are and the water balance of your body.

Be realistic! Don't set your goals too high. A loss of one

to two pounds each week is a success story! Anticipate plateaus, because virtually everyone involved in a weight-control program has his or her ups and downs. And should you at some point yield to temptation and devour an extra helping of turkey and dressing, don't despair—just don't make a habit of it. After all, we have all, on occasion, fallen off the wagon.

* * *

We've talked some in this book about "behavior modification," a system based on the behaviorist principles of B. F. Skinner. This system has been highly successful in the treatment of a variety of problems—from overeating to anxiety. In fact, almost all the suggestions and techniques so far outlined in this book—from keeping a record of your eating habits to avoiding locations in your home which may trigger an impulse to snack—are based on behavior-modification techniques. Even your new exercise program is based on this technique.

The key to behavior modification—whether the system is applied to former smokers who do not want to gain weight or to people suffering from psychological disorders—is that small changes in behavior eventually lead to greater changes. Each step leads to a final goal. What is most important is that you, the new ex-smoker, be aware that you can change your life and remain determined to do so.

As you already have learned, there are dozens of changes you can make in your lifestyle to survive as an ex-smoker and avoid putting on pounds as well. The following list contains even more suggestions to help you attain that goal:

1. Have a glass of water, club soda, tea, or diet cola twenty minutes before eating. It will help take the edge off your appetite.
2. Never skip meals—especially breakfast. Avoid the practice of having little or no lunch and a big dinner.

3. When you eat, concentrate. Remain aware of what you're eating and how much. Don't do anything else while eating.

4. Try using only one hand to eat with. This keeps you from grabbing other foods and forces you to eat more slowly.

5. If you get into an argument or become angry—don't eat. Have a glass of water instead.

6. Instead of eating candy while driving, sing along with the radio.

7. Freeze foods that tempt you. If you have to thaw them out, it will help prevent compulsive eating.

8. So as not to tempt yourself, store food in opaque containers, metal cannisters, coffee cans, or any other type of container you cannot see through.

9. When eating out, plan what you want to eat before entering a restaurant. This will prevent fattening menu temptations.

10. Eat only when you are really hungry. Learn the difference between true hunger and appetite signals.

11. If you don't know what you want to eat, then you're not really hungry.

12. Eat one food at a time in order of preference.

13. Try to put aside a portion of the food you like the least during a meal. Gradually put aside small portions of other foods and side dishes.

14. Drink six ten-ounce glasses of water a day. Experts say it keeps you hydrated. If your body cells are not hydrated, they are unable to properly burn off fat. Water is also good for removing any toxins due to the weight reduction process and, in many people, reducing the desire to smoke.

15. Think carefully about that piece of pie which is tempting you so. View it as a substance made of hydrogenated fat, refined sugar, and white flour. See it not as a tempting treat, but something unwholesome to put into your body.

16. Take a break during a meal. Get up from the table and get a glass of water. Use this time to reflect on your reasons for wanting to maintain or lose weight.

17. Split a single slice of bread into two slices for a sandwich.

18. Don't use food as a companion. When you're feeling lonely or bored, turn to a friend—not to a slice of cherry pie.

19. Since the evening hours are the most dangerous times for food bingeing or snacking temptations, try not to be alone at night for a while.

20. Keep a good stock of diet soda or juices on hand for between-meal emergencies.

21. Never eat alone if you can help it.

22. Cooking is a problem time. Whenever you stir the pot you may like to take a taste. Allow yourself only one taste and then get some other member of your family to stir the pot.

23. Bake on a full stomach so you won't be tempted.

24. Post signs around your kitchen which remind you of your goals.

25. Weigh yourself each morning. Reward yourself if you've lost weight.

26. If you're going to a party, tell your friends in advance that you're dieting. This will lessen your chances of cheating, because you don't want to show your friends that you have no willpower.

27. Feeling anxious or stressful? Busy your hands, not your mouth.

28. If you're alone and you feel like snacking, set a three-minute egg timer. Tell yourself that you will wait at least three minutes before succumbing to temptation. Now think about what you're planning to do.

29. Poach, soft-boil, or hard-boil your eggs.

30. Remember: Beginning a diet is not beginning a prison sentence. You don't have to deny yourself all the foods you've always loved. Just eat fewer of them and in smaller amounts.

The following chart contains the latest government recommendations on the range of acceptable weight. The table gives you an idea of the ideal weight based on age and height, but does not spell out which end of the weight range is right for you. Figures apply to men and women.

	Age				
Height	*20–29*	*30–39*	*40–49*	*50–59*	*60–69*
4'10"	84–111	92–119	99–127	107–135	115–142
4'11"	87–115	95–123	103–131	111–139	119–147
5'	90–119	98–127	106–135	114–143	123–152
5'1"	93–123	101–131	110–140	118–148	127–157
5'2"	96–127	105–136	113–144	122–153	131–163
5'3"	99–131	108–140	117–149	126–158	135–168
5'4"	102–135	112–145	121–154	130–163	140–173
5'5"	106–140	115–149	125–159	134–168	144–179
5'6"	109–144	119–154	129–164	138–174	148–184
5'7"	112–148	122–159	133–169	143–179	153–190
5'8"	116–153	126–163	137–174	147–184	158–196
5'9"	119–157	130–168	141–179	151–190	162–201
5'10"	122–162	134–173	145–184	156–195	167–207
5'11"	126–167	137–178	149–190	160–201	172–213
6'	129–171	141–183	153–195	165–207	177–219
6'1"	133–176	145–188	157–200	169–213	182–225
6'2"	137–181	149–194	162–206	174–219	187–232
6'3"	141–186	153–199	166–212	179–225	192–238
6'4"	144–191	157–205	171–218	184–231	197–244

E·L·E·V·E·N

A POCKET FULL OF MIRACLES

The new ex-smoker who may be experiencing some problems with weight gain is likely to take the bait offered by one of the many so-called "miracle diets"—those quickie diets that promise a slimmer you in thirty days or less.

The truth of the matter, however, is that these diets rarely work. Like Hula-Hoops, toga parties, and miniskirts, they come and go, leaving you unchanged in the pounds column.

Not only do government studies of many of these popular diets cast grave doubt on whether they are as successful as they claim to be, but in some cases researchers have found the diets to be so nutritionally unbalanced that they could be harmful to you if followed for a long period of time.

So be leery of those miracle diets which promise quick results, particularly if they encourage eating little or no food. Fasting is especially dangerous because it breaks down muscle as well as fat and this puts a tremendous strain on the liver and kidneys. The result can be weakness, faintness, headaches, and nausea. Don't try any fasting program unless it is recommended and supervised by your physician.

Many popular diet fads encourage people to avoid food which contains carbohydrates. But according to researchers, eliminating carbohydrates from your diet can lead to a condition called ketosis. Ketosis does cause rapid weight loss, but those pounds you shed are mostly water. People in a ketotic state can lose their appetite and become weak, fatigued, dehydrated, and nauseated. Fortunately, these symptoms usually disappear when a balanced diet containing carbohydrates is resumed, but you will also gain back the water weight which you lost while on the diet.

Before you try any reducing diet you've read or heard about, make sure it's nutritionally sound. We're now going to show you some ways to evaluate a diet, but if you're still not sure check with your doctor, dietitian, or health department nutritionist. Also, you might want to check *Consumer Guide,* which frequently rates diets and suggests which are the best.

When considering a diet, first carefully read the specific diet plan and then ask yourself the following questions. If you answer yes to all of them, you've probably found a weight-reducing program that's good for you.

1. Are there fewer calories in this weight-loss diet than in food you normally eat? Remember, you only lose weight by reducing your caloric intake below your energy output.

2. Does the plan include a variety of foods from these groups: fruit, vegetable; bread, cereal; milk, cheese; meat, poultry, fish, and dried beans? It's important to have foods from each of these groups in your diet every day.

3. Is the plan made up of appealing food that you will enjoy eating, not just for several weeks or months but for the rest of your life?

4. Are the foods available at the grocery store where you usually shop? If products are not easily available, you may end up losing interest in the diet. Unusual foods are sometimes obtainable only at specialty stores and often cost more than regular foods.

5. Does the diet allow you to eat some of your favorite foods occasionally? On a sensible diet program there's room for a rich dessert in small amounts once in a while.

6. Does the diet recommend changes in your eating habits that also fit your lifestyle and pocketbook?

Let's now examine some of the more popular diets that are being heavily promoted across the country, today, and some of the problems they present.

One of the most popular diets calls for unlimited protein and little or no carbohydrates. The diet recommends that you concentrate on eating lean meat, poultry, fish, eggs, and low-fat cheeses. It also suggests that you drink at least eight ten-ounce glasses of water a day in addition to coffee, tea, diet soda, or alcohol.

The problem with this diet is that only protein-rich foods are emphasized. Essential vitamins and minerals, along with variety, are missing. This diet quickly loses appeal. In addition, blood cholesterol level may increase due to a high intake of saturated fat and cholesterol. This diet will lead to a ketotic condition, which we've discussed earlier.

A second popular diet stresses unlimited protein and fat, and some carbohydrates. You are supposed to eat as much as you want of foods rich in protein and fat (this is said to cause the body to burn fat). You are also asked to gradually increase your consumption of carbohydrate foods to forty grams to maintain your weight.

This plan emphasizes foods that are high in saturated fat

and cholesterol. Thus, adhering to this diet may cause an increase in your blood cholesterol level. Essential vitamins and minerals are lacking. You may find yourself eating foods with more calories than you can use, and these excess calories may cause weight gain rather than loss over a period of time. You may also develop a state of ketosis.

A third popular diet recommends liquid protein or supplemented fasting. This diet is promoted as a means of burning off fat while sparing muscle. Without additional food, this diet provides only 300 to 500 calories per day.

Such diets are considered by researchers to be nutritionally incomplete. Muscle breakdown may occur, and in addition nausea, vomiting, diarrhea, constipation, faintness, muscle cramps, and fatigue may result. This diet could be potentially dangerous, especially for people with kidney, liver, and heart diseases, and for the elderly. Some deaths have been reported in association with this diet.

There are also many popular low-calorie, high-fiber diets on the market. Highly refined and processed foods are eliminated and, instead, whole grains, raw fruits and vegetables, and nuts and seeds are emphasized. The diet also calls for small-to-moderate amounts of lean meat. Poultry and fish are allowed, but very little fat.

The low-calorie, high-fiber diet can sometimes pose problems because it can irritate the intestinal tract until the body adjusts to fiber intake. Its acceptance by the body may be a problem because of the high amount of roughage and the small amount of fat and lean meat, poultry, and fish. This diet, which calls for a maximum of 600 calories per day, is nutritionally inadequate.

Finally, there is a quite popular diet which suggests high protein with fructose as a major carbohydrate. In this diet, sugar (sucrose) is replaced by specific amounts of fructose (crystals, flavored tablets, and liquids) on the premise that fructose will appease the appetite. Five servings (about 800 calories) of meat, poultry, fish, and eggs, plus two large salads make up daily meals. Beverages sweetened with fructose are encouraged.

This diet is nutritionally unbalanced because no foods from the milk-cheese or bread-cereal groups are included. And using fructose as a sweetener does not retrain you to enjoy less sweet foods. Fructose, by the way, has as many calories per gram as sugar; however, fructose is supposed to taste sweeter, so less may be used. Also, there is no evidence that fructose affects your appetite for sweets, and it may also cause undesirable increases in triglyceride (a fat component) levels in the blood.

There are many other weight-loss methods—from bypass surgery where the stomach is greatly reduced in size to jaw wiring—and you should view all these methods with a healthy dose of skepticism. There is no pocket full of miracles—no magical pills—when it comes to weight loss. The best diet plan—whether you're attempting to shed extra pounds or just trying to stay healthy—is a well-balanced one.

This may be the appropriate time to offer a few tips about healthful eating. It's important that you assure yourself an adequate diet, especially now when your body is going through a critical readjustment period.

You need about forty different nutrients to stay healthy, and the simplest rule of thumb to make sure that you get your proper quota of nutrients—these include vitamins, minerals, and essential fatty and amino acids—is to eat a variety of foods. No single food item supplies all the essential nutrients in the amounts that you need.

One way to assure variety along with a well-balanced diet is to select foods each day from each of several major groups: for example, fruits and vegetables; cereals, breads, and grains; meats, poultry, eggs, and fish; dried peas and beans and black-eyed peas, which are good vegetable sources of protein; and milk, cheese, and yogurt.

Fruits and vegetables are excellent sources of vitamins—especially vitamins C and A. Whole-grain and enriched breads, cereals, and grain products provide B vitamins, iron, and energy. Meats supply protein, fat, iron, and other minerals, as well as several vitamins, including thiamine and vitamin B_{12}. Dairy products are major sources of calcium and other nutrients.

Try to eat less fat and more carbohydrates, because excess fat is a major source of excess calories. You should avoid saturated fats in such foods as beef, pork, butter, cream, whole milk, and ice cream. On the other hand, polyunsaturated fat, such as that found in fish, most vegetable oils (except coconut oil), pecans, walnuts, and most margarines, are good for you. Also avoid too much cholesterol and salt.

Remember that when you cut down on the amount of saturated fats in your daily diet, you can increase the number of complex carbohydrates—from foods such as whole-grain breads, cereals, beans, and vegetables—without gaining any weight. The worst offenders in terms of weight gain are simple carbohydrates such as sugar.

We've said it before, but we'll say it again. If you want to lose weight, do so gradually. A steady loss of one to two pounds a week—until you reach your goal—is relatively safe, and more likely to be maintained than a more drastic reduction. Long-term success depends upon acquiring new and better habits of eating and exercise, which is why "crash" diets usually fail in the long run.

Above all, stay away from those crash diets that are severely restricted in the variety of foods they allow. Diets containing fewer than 800 calories may also be hazardous to your health.

Menu Ideas

Here are some menu ideas (courtesy of the American Dietetic Association) that are ideal for a day in the life of an ex-smoker or anyone who is following the low-calorie trail. These menus, which meet or exceed the Recommended Dietary Allowances for most nutrients, show you how you might combine foods that are pleasing and nutritious, while low in calories. The calorie count ranges from 1,800 down to 1,200.

1,800-Calorie Menu

BREAKFAST

¾ cup orange juice

1 poached egg

2 bran muffins

2 teaspoons margarine

1 cup skim milk

LUNCH

1 cup split pea soup

Chicken salad sandwich (½ cup chicken salad, made with low-calorie mayonnaise-type salad dressing; 2 slices rye bread)

2 small pear halves, canned in light sirup

Water, tea, or coffee

DINNER

1 serving sweet and sour pork chops

1 small baked sweet potato

½ cup broccoli, cooked

⅔ cup fruit cup (apples, oranges, bananas)

1 whole-wheat roll

1 teaspoon margarine

Water, tea, or coffee

SNACK

1 cup skim milk

4 whole-wheat crackers

1,500-Calorie Menu

BREAKFAST

½ cup grapefruit juice, unsweetened

1 shredded wheat biscuit

1 slice whole-wheat toast

1 teaspoon margarine

½ cup skim milk

LUNCH

Roast beef sandwich (3 ounces cooked, lean roast beef, 1 lettuce leaf, 2 teaspoons mayonnaise-type salad dressing, 2 slices whole-wheat bread)

6 to 8 carrot strips (2½"–3" long)

1 medium orange

Water, tea, or coffee

DINNER

1 serving baked fish fillet

1 baked potato

2 teaspoons margarine

½ cup green peas, cooked

Salad (½ tomato, sliced, ½ cucumber, sliced, 2 tablespoons yogurt dressing)

1 medium slice French bread

1 teaspoon margarine

½ cup peach slices, fresh

Water, tea, or coffee

SNACK

¾ cup plain lowfat yogurt

¼ cup blueberries, fresh or frozen (unsweetened)

1,200-Calorie Menu

BREAKFAST

¾ cup bran flakes

¾ cup strawberries, fresh

¾ cup plain lowfat yogurt

LUNCH

1 serving chef's salad

2 tablespoons salad dressing, Italian, regular

4 rye wafers

1 medium tangerine

Water, tea, or coffee

DINNER

1 serving beef Stroganoff (with noodles)

½ cup spinach, cooked

1 whole-wheat roll

1 teaspoon margarine

¼ cantaloupe, 5-inch diameter

1 cup skim milk

SNACK

1 medium banana

Recipes

In the following pages you will find a variety of recipes for foods that are lower in calories, fat, sugar, and salt than most similar ones you may find in many cookbooks. Use these recipes as a guide to alter your favorite—but fattening—dishes to fit into a balanced, health-promoting diet.

All the following recipes have been supplied courtesy of the American Dietetic Association. The recipes were developed in United States Department of Agriculture laboratories to give a reasonable return in nutrients for the calories supplied. All the recipes have been taste-panel tested and are light in calories. They call for skim and low-fat milk and dairy products, lean cuts of meat, lean fish and poultry.

Because not every dish suggested here may be suitable for your diet plan, we have included a list estimating the caloric, fat, and cholesterol contents so that you can determine for yourself whether such a meal is right for your diet.

Soups

MANHATTAN CHICKEN CHOWDER

Four servings, 1 cup each
Per serving:
    Calories: 135
    Total fat: 3.0 grams

Saturated fat: 0.8 gram
Cholesterol: 43 milligrams

½ cup carrots, chopped
½ cup celery, chopped
½ cup turnips, diced
¼ cup onion, chopped
¼ teaspoon salt
1 cup chicken broth
1 16-ounce can tomatoes
⅛ teaspoon thyme leaves
⅛ teaspoon pepper
1½ cups chicken, cooked, diced

---

1. Add carrots, celery, turnips, onion, and salt to boiling chicken broth. Cover and boil gently until vegetables are tender, about 10 minutes.
2. Break up large pieces of tomato.
3. Add tomatoes, thyme, pepper, and chicken to cooked vegetables.
4. Simmer, covered, 10 minutes to blend flavors.

√ *Menu Suggestion:* Serve with rye crackers. Have fresh pear wedges for dessert.

VEGETABLE SOUP

Four servings, about 1 cup each
Per serving:
Calories: 65.
Total fat: 0.4 gram
Saturated fat: trace
Cholesterol: 0

171

¼ cup onion, chopped
½ cup celery, diced
½ cup carrots, sliced
½ cup potatoes, diced
½ cup cabbage, shredded
½ cup turnips, diced
1 tablespoon parsley, chopped
½ cup frozen cut green beans
¼ teaspoon basil leaves
⅛ teaspoon pepper
1 bay leaf
1½ cups boiling water
1 16-ounce can tomatoes

1. Add all ingredients except tomatoes to boiling water. Cover and boil gently 15 minutes.
2. Break up large pieces of tomato.
3. Add tomatoes to vegetable mixture and continue cooking until vegetables are tender, about 20 minutes.
4. Remove bay leaf.

SPINACH SOUP

Four servings, about 1 cup each
Per serving:

Calories: 105
Total fat: 3.2 grams
Saturated fat: 0.7 gram
Cholesterol: 2 milligrams

---

1 10-ounce package frozen chopped spinach
¼ cup carrots, shredded
¼ cup celery, chopped
2 tablespoons onion, chopped
½ teaspoon dill weed
1 cup boiling water
¼ teaspoon salt
2 cups skim milk
1 tablespoon margarine
2 tablespoons flour
3 tablespoons water

---

1. Add vegetables and dill weed to boiling salted water. Cover and boil gently until vegetables are tender, about 15 minutes.
2. Stir in spinach.
3. Add milk and margarine. Heat to simmering.
4. Mix flour with 3 tablespoons water until smooth. Add slowly to vegetable mixture, stirring constantly. Heat until mixture just starts to boil.

Entrees

ITALIAN FISH ROLLUPS

Four servings, 1 rollup each
Per serving:
Calories: 125 with flounder; 120 with cod
Total fat: 1.5 grams
Saturated fat: 0.5 gram
Cholesterol: 51 milligrams with flounder; 46 milligrams with cod

1 pound flounder or cod fillets, fresh or frozen, without skin

1 9-ounce package frozen French-style green beans

2 tablespoons onion, chopped

½ cup boiling water

1 8-ounce can tomato sauce

¼ teaspoon oregano leaves

¼ teaspoon basil leaves

⅛ teaspoon garlic powder

1 tablespoon grated Parmesan cheese

1. Thaw frozen fish in refrigerator overnight. Divide fish into four servings.

2. Add beans and onion to boiling water. Cover and boil gently until beans are tender but still crisp—about 7 minutes. Drain.

3. Place one-quarter of the bean-onion mixture in the middle of each fish portion.

4. Start with narrow end of fillet and roll. Place in baking pan with ends of fillets underneath.

5. Mix tomato sauce, oregano, basil, and garlic powder. Pour over fish rollups.

6. Sprinkle with cheese.

7. Bake at 350°F. (moderate oven) until fish flakes easily when tested with a fork, about 45 minutes.

√ *Menu Suggestion:* Serve with yellow summer squash and bran muffins.

BAKED FISH FILLETS

Four servings, about 3 ounces each

Per serving:

Calories: 115

Total fat: 3.2 grams

Saturated fat: 0.7 gram
Cholesterol: 60 milligrams

---

1 pound fresh or frozen ocean perch fillets
2 teaspoons margarine, melted
1 tablespoon lemon juice
½ teaspoon salt
¼ teaspoon paprika
1 teaspoon parsley, chopped

---

1. Thaw frozen fish in refrigerator overnight.
2. Lightly grease a shallow baking pan. Place fillets in a single layer, skin side down, in pan.
3. Mix margarine, lemon juice, salt, and paprika. Spoon over fillets.
4. Bake at 350°F. (moderate oven) until fish flakes easily when tested with a fork, about 20 minutes.
5. Garnish each serving with parsley.

√ *Menu Suggestion:* Serve with herbed broccoli and tomato-cucumber salad.

BAKED STEAK WITH CREOLE SAUCE

Four servings, about 2¼ ounces each
Per serving:
    Calories: 190
    Total fat: 7.7 grams
    Saturated fat: 2.9 grams
    Cholesterol: 74 milligrams

¼ cup onion, chopped
¼ cup green pepper, chopped
2 teaspoons oil

1 8-ounce can tomatoes
¼ teaspoon salt
⅛ teaspoon pepper
1 pound beef round steak, boneless

---

1. Cook onion and green pepper in oil until onion is clear.
2. Break up large pieces of tomato.
3. Add tomatoes, salt, and pepper to cooked onion and green pepper.
4. Cover and simmer 20 minutes to blend flavors.
5. Trim fat from steak.
6. Brown steak lightly on both sides in hot frying pan. Place in baking pan.
7. Pour sauce over steak.
8. Cover and bake at 350°F. (moderate oven) until steak is tender, about 1½ hours.

√ *Menu Suggestion:* Serve with whole green beans and parsleyed potatoes.

BAKED STUFFED FISH

Four servings, about 3 ounces fish each

Per serving:

   Calories: 185
   Total fat: 5.6 grams with haddock; 5.8 grams with cod
   Saturated fat: 1.0 gram
   Cholesterol: 69 milligrams with haddock; 57 milligrams with cod

---

1 pound haddock or cod fillets, fresh or frozen, without skin
2 teaspoons oil
¼ cup onion, chopped

¼ cup celery, chopped

2 cups whole-wheat bread cubes, soft

4 teaspoons parsley, chopped

¼ teaspoon sage

¼ teaspoon salt

⅛ teaspoon pepper

1 tablespoon margarine, melted

―――――――――

1. Thaw frozen fish in refrigerator overnight.
2. Heat oil in small frying pan. Add onion and celery. Cover and cook, stirring.
3. Stir in bread cubes, 3 teaspoons of parsley, sage, salt, and pepper.
4. Arrange half of fillets in a lightly oiled, shallow baking pan. Spread bread mixture over fillets in pan. Top with remaining fillets.
5. Cover and bake at 325°F. (slow oven) for 15 minutes.
6. Mix margarine with remaining parsley. Spoon over fish fillets. Continue baking, uncovered, until fish flakes easily when tested with a fork, about 10 minutes.

√ *Menu Suggestion:* Serve with seasoned kale and sliced tomatoes on salad greens.

―――――――――

BEEF BURGUNDY

Four servings, about 1 cup each

Per serving:

    Calories: 225
    Total fat: 4.3 grams
    Saturated fat: 1.9 grams
    Cholesterol: 55 milligrams

―――――――――

¾ pound beef round, well-trimmed, cut into 1-inch cubes.

½ teaspoon salt

⅛ teaspoon pepper

1 bay leaf

⅛ teaspoon thyme leaves

1½ cups water

1½ cups potatoes, diced

1 cup carrots, sliced

½ cup celery, diced

⅓ cup onion, chopped

1 cup fresh mushrooms, sliced

3 tablespoons flour

¼ cup water

⅓ cup red burgundy wine

Parsley, to garnish

---

1. Brown beef cubes in hot frying pan.
2. Add salt, pepper, bay leaf, thyme, and 1½ cups water.
3. Simmer, covered, until beef is almost tender, about 1¾ hours.
4. Remove bay leaf.
5. Add potatoes, carrots, celery, onion, and mushrooms. Simmer, covered, until vegetables are tender, about 20 minutes.
6. Mix flour with ¼ cup water until smooth. Add slowly to meat mixture, stirring gently. Cook until thickened.
7. Stir in wine.
8. Garnish with parsley.

√ *Menu Suggestion:* Serve on a small bed of noodles. Have fresh fruit for dessert.

CHICKEN AND ZUCCHINI

Four servings, about ⅔ cup each

Per serving:

    Calories: 125
    Total fat: 3.7 grams
    Saturated fat: 0.4 gram
    Cholesterol: 51 milligrams

---

3 chicken breast halves, boneless, without skin
2 teaspoons oil
1 clove garlic, cut in quarters
1 tablespoon soy sauce
⅓ cup celery, thinly sliced
1 2-ounce can mushroom slices, drained
1 cup zucchini squash, cut into thin strips
2 teaspoons cornstarch
3 tablespoons water

---

1. Slice chicken into thin strips, about ⅛ inch wide. (It is easier to slice chicken thinly if it is partially frozen.)
2. Heat oil in nonstick frying pan. Add chicken and garlic.
3. Cook, stirring constantly, until chicken turns white, about 5 minutes. Remove garlic pieces.
4. Stir in soy sauce.
5. Add celery, mushrooms, and squash.
6. Cook, covered, until vegetables are tender-crisp, about 4 minutes.
7. Mix cornstarch with water until smooth. Add slowly to chicken mixture, stirring constantly.
8. Continue cooking until ingredients are coated with a thin glaze, about 1 minute.

√ *Menu Suggestion:* Serve with broiled tomatoes. Have a fruit cup for dessert.

CURRIED PORK

Four servings, about ½ cup curry and ½ cup rice each

Per serving:
   Calories: 250
   Total fat: 5.6 grams
   Saturated fat: 1.5 grams
   Cholesterol: 32 milligrams

¼ cup onion, chopped

2 cups tart apple, unpared, chopped

1 tablespoon oil

2 tablespoons flour

½ teaspoon salt

⅛ teaspoon ground ginger

1 teaspoon curry powder

1 cup skim milk

1 cup pork, cooked, diced

2 cups brown rice, cooked, unsalted

---

1. Cook onion and apple in oil until tender.

2. Stir in flour, salt, ginger, and curry powder.

3. Add milk slowly, stirring constantly. Cook until thickened.

4. Add pork. Heat to serving temperature.

5. Serve over rice.

√ *Menu Suggestion:* Serve with a small green salad with yogurt dressing. Have a ginger wheat cookie for dessert.

DENVER-STYLE SCRAMBLED EGGS

Four servings, about ⅓ cup each

Per serving:

Calories: 130
Total fat: 8.2 grams
Saturated fat: 2.5 grams
Cholesterol: 290 milligrams

---

2 teaspoons onion, very finely chopped
1 tablespoon green pepper, very finely chopped
1 teaspoon margarine
¼ cup skim milk
4 eggs, slightly beaten
⅛ teaspoon salt
Dash pepper
½ cup pork, cooked, chopped
2 teaspoons pimiento, finely chopped
2 teaspoons parsley, chopped

---

1. Cook onion and green pepper in margarine in covered nonstick frying pan until tender.
2. Mix milk, eggs, salt, and pepper. Beat until frothy.
3. Pour egg mixture into pan with onion and green pepper.
4. Cook, stirring occasionally, until eggs begin to set.
5. Stir in pork, pimiento, and parsley.
6. Cook until eggs are set.

√ *Menu Suggestion:* Serve with whole-wheat toast and citrus fruit cup.

FLANK STEAK ORIENTAL

Four servings, about 2½ ounces each

Per serving:

Calories: 185 with sherry; 175 without sherry
Total fat: 7.8 grams
Saturated fat: 3.0 grams
Cholesterol: 71 milligrams

---

2 tablespoons oil
1 tablespoon vinegar
1 tablespoon soy sauce
¼ cup sherry (see note below)
1 tablespoon honey
1 tablespoon onion, very finely chopped
1 clove garlic, cut in quarters
½ teaspoon ground ginger
1 pound flank steak

---

1. The day before serving, mix all ingredients except the steak.
2. Place steak in shallow dish. Pour oil mixture over steak. Cover and refrigerate 18 to 24 hours, turning steak over several times.
3. The day of serving, remove steak and garlic pieces from oil mixture. Discard garlic.
4. Place steak on broiler pan. Brush with oil mixture.
5. Broil about 2 inches from heat, allowing about 7 minutes per side. Brush with oil mixture when steak is turned.
6. To serve, slice into thin slices, cutting across the grain on the diagonal from top to bottom of the steak.

√ *Menu Suggestion:* Serve with fluffy rice and snow peas.

Note: Sherry may be omitted if desired. Increase vinegar to 2 tablespoons and add 1 tablespoon Worcestershire sauce and 2 tablespoons water to other ingredients.

INDIVIDUAL MEAT LOAVES

Four servings, 1 loaf each

Per serving:

Calories: 200
Total fat: 9.8 grams
Saturated fat: 4.4 grams
Cholesterol: 137 milligrams

¾ pound ground beef, extra lean
1 egg
¼ cup skim milk
¼ cup onion, finely chopped
½ cup breadcrumbs, soft
¼ teaspoon salt
Dash pepper
Dash sage

---

1. Mix ground beef with other ingredients.
2. Shape into 4 loaves. Place in an 8-by-8-by-2-inch baking pan.
3. Bake at 350°F. (moderate oven) until loaves are done in the center, about 40 minutes.

√ *Menu Suggestion:* Serve with mashed potatoes and assorted fresh vegetable sticks.

LEMON BAKED CHICKEN

Four servings, 1 chicken breast half each

Per serving:

Calories: 190
Total fat: 9.1 grams

Saturated fat: 1.9 grams
Cholesterol: 60 milligrams

---

3 tablespoons lemon juice

2 tablespoons oil

1 tablespoon onion, very finely chopped

¼ teaspoon salt

⅛ teaspoon paprika

4 chicken breast halves, boneless, without skin

---

1. Mix all ingredients except chicken.

2. Place chicken pieces in shallow baking pan.

3. Mix lemon juice, oil, onion, salt, and paprika together and pour mixture over chicken pieces.

4. Bake at 400°F. (hot oven) until chicken is tender, about 1 hour. Baste chicken several times with liquid in pan during baking.

√ *Menu Suggestion:* Serve with baked potato and green peas.

MOCK BEEF STROGANOFF

Four servings, ½ cup stroganoff and ⅓ cup noodles each

Per serving:

Calories: 220
Total fat: 4.9 grams
Saturated fat: 2 grams
Cholesterol: 70 milligrams

¾ pound beef round steak, boneless

¼ pound fresh mushrooms

½ cup onion, sliced

½ cup beef broth, condensed

½ cup water

1 tablespoon catsup

⅛ teaspoon pepper

2 tablespoons flour

1 cup buttermilk

1⅓ cups (about 1¾ cups uncooked) noodles, cooked, unsalted

---

1. Trim all fat from steak. Slice steak across the grain into thin strips, about ⅛ inch wide and 3 inches long. (It is easier to slice meat thinly if it is partially frozen.)

2. Wash and slice mushrooms.

3. Cook beef strips, mushrooms, and onion in a nonstick frying pan until beef is lightly browned.

4. Add broth, water, catsup, and pepper. Cover and simmer until beef is tender, about 45 minutes.

5. Mix flour with about ¼ cup of the buttermilk until smooth. Add remaining buttermilk. Stir into beef mixture. Cook, stirring constantly, until thickened.

6. Serve over noodles.

√ *Menu Suggestion:* Serve with a tossed green salad.

STIR-FRIED BEEF WITH VEGETABLES

Four servings, about ¾ cup each

Per serving:

Calories: 210 with sherry; 190 with broth
Total fat: 8.5 grams
Saturated fat: 2.6 grams
Cholesterol: 55 milligrams with sherry; 57 milligrams with broth

---

¾ pound beef round steak, boneless
4 teaspoons oil
⅓ cup carrots, in ⅛-inch diagonal slices
⅓ cup onion, sliced
⅓ cup celery, in ⅛-inch diagonal slices
2 cups fresh mung bean sprouts
½ tablespoon cornstarch
½ teaspoon ground ginger
⅛ teaspoon garlic powder
1 tablespoon soy sauce
¼ cup sherry (see note below)

---

1. Trim all fat from steak. Slice steak across the grain into thin strips, about ⅛ inch wide and 3 inches long. (It is easier to slice meat thinly if it is partially frozen.)
2. Heat 2 teaspoons of the oil in frying pan. Add beef strips and stir-fry over moderately high heat, turning pieces constantly until beef is no longer red, about 2 to 3 minutes.
3. Remove beef from frying pan.
4. Heat remaining 2 teaspoons of oil in frying pan. Add carrots. Stir-fry 1 minute.
5. Add onion, celery, and bean sprouts. Continue to stir-fry until vegetables are tender-crisp, about 3 to 4 minutes.
6. Mix cornstarch, ginger, and garlic powder with soy sauce and sherry until smooth. Add slowly to vegetables, stirring constantly. Continue cooking until bubbly.
7. Stir in beef.
8. Reduce heat and cook, covered, 1 minute.

Note: Sherry may be omitted if desired. Use ¼ cup beef broth in place of sherry.

√ *Menu Suggestion:* Serve with brown rice. Have fresh peach slices for dessert.

SWEET-SOUR PORK CHOPS

Four servings, 1 chop with ⅓ cup sauce each
Per serving:
    Calories: 185
    Total fat: 7.4 grams
    Saturated fat: 2.6 grams
    Cholesterol: 38 milligrams

4 (about 1 pound) loin pork chops, thin cut
1 tablespoon cornstarch
¼ cup vinegar
½ cup pineapple juice (and water if needed)
1 tablespoon soy sauce
1 tablespoon brown sugar, packed
1 small green pepper, cut in squares
1 cup canned pineapple chunks in natural juice, drained

1. Trim fat from pork chops.
2. Brown pork chops on both sides in nonstick frying pan.
3. Mix cornstarch with vinegar until smooth. Add juice and water mixture, soy sauce, and sugar. Cook over low heat. Stir constantly until thickened.
4. Pour sauce over pork chops.
5. Simmer, covered, until pork chops are almost tender, about 30 minutes.
6. Add green pepper and pineapple.

7. Simmer, covered, until pork chops are tender and green pepper is tender-crisp, about 10 minutes longer.

√ *Menu Suggestion:* Serve with seasoned spinach.

TURKEY (OR CHICKEN) DIVAN

Four servings, about ¾ cup each

Per serving:

Calories: 175 with turkey; 170 with chicken
Total fat: 5.2 grams with turkey; 5 grams with chicken
Saturated fat: 2.4 grams
Cholesterol: 53 milligrams with turkey; 54 milligrams with chicken

---

1 10-ounce package frozen broccoli spears
8 ounces turkey (or chicken) breast, cooked, sliced
2 tablespoons cornstarch
½ cup turkey broth, unsalted
½ cup skim milk
⅓ cup natural cheddar cheese, shredded
¼ teaspoon salt

---

1. Cook broccoli as directed on package until just tender. Drain.
2. Arrange broccoli in 1½-quart casserole. Lay turkey slices on top of broccoli.
3. Mix cornstarch with broth in saucepan until smooth. Add milk. Cook, stirring constantly, until thickened. Remove from heat.
4. Add cheese and salt. Stir until cheese melts.
5. Pour sauce over turkey.
6. Bake at 375°F. (moderate oven) until sauce is bubbly, about 25 minutes.

√ *Menu Suggestion:* Serve with a peach-blueberry salad.

Vegetables

SQUASH-BROCCOLI MEDLEY

Four servings, about ½ cup each
Per serving:
  Calories: 40
  Total fat: 3.0 grams
  Saturated fat: 0.5 gram
  Cholesterol: 0

½ cup fresh mushrooms, sliced
1 tablespoon margarine
1 cup fresh broccoli, cut in 1-inch pieces
1 cup yellow summer squash, sliced
1 cup zucchini squash, sliced
¼ teaspoon salt
⅛ teaspoon pepper
½ cup water
¼ teaspoon lemon rind, grated

---

1. Cook mushrooms in margarine in nonstick frying pan until lightly browned.
2. Add remaining ingredients except lemon rind.
3. Cover and boil gently until vegetables are tender, about 10 minutes. Drain.
4. Gently stir in lemon rind.

DILLED ZUCCHINI SQUASH

Four servings, ½ cup each

Per serving:

   Calories: 15
   Total fat: 0.1 gram
   Saturated fat: trace
   Cholesterol: 0

---

1 pound zucchini squash

⅓ cup onion, chopped

¼ cup boiling water

⅛ teaspoon salt

½ teaspoon paprika

½ teaspoon dill weed

1 tablespoon vinegar

---

1. Remove ends from squash. Cut into strips or slices.
2. Add squash and onion to boiling, salted water. Cover and boil gently until tender, about 10 minutes. Drain.
3. Add paprika, dill weed, and vinegar. Stir gently.

MASHED POTATO PATTIES

Four servings, 2 patties each

Per serving:

   Calories: 80
   Total fat: 2.4 grams
   Saturated fat: 0.6 gram
   Cholesterol: 69 milligrams

1½ cups mashed potatoes (see note below)

1 egg, beaten

2 teaspoons chives, finely chopped

¼ teaspoon salt
Dash pepper
1 teaspoon margarine

---

1. Mix potatoes, egg, chives, salt, and pepper well. Shape into 8 patties.
2. Melt margarine in nonstick frying pan. Cook patties over low heat until lightly browned, about 5 minutes on each side.

Note: Mashed potatoes should be made using skim milk. Omit margarine.

HERBED BROCCOLI

Four servings, about ½ cup each
Per serving:
   Calories: 20
   Total fat: 0.2 gram
   Saturated fat: 0
   Cholesterol: 0

¾ pound fresh broccoli spears
2 teaspoons onion, finely chopped
½ teaspoon marjoram leaves
½ teaspoon basil leaves
¾ cup boiling water
4 lemon wedges

---

1. Wash and trim broccoli. Split thick stems.
2. Add broccoli, onion, and herbs to boiling water.

3. Cover and boil gently until broccoli is tender, about 10 minutes. Drain.

4. Serve with lemon wedge garnish.

Note: A 10-ounce package frozen broccoli spears may be used in place of fresh broccoli. Cook frozen broccoli about 6 minutes. Servings will be slightly smaller.

SEASONED GREEN BEANS

Four servings, about ½ cup each

Per serving:

    Calories: 40
    Total fat: 1.1 grams
    Saturated fat: 0.2 gram
    Cholesterol: 0

¼ cup onion, chopped

¼ cup celery, chopped

1 teaspoon margarine

3 cups frozen cut green beans

⅛ teaspoon garlic powder

⅛ teaspoon salt

Dash pepper

¼ cup water

1. Cook onion and celery in margarine in nonstick frying pan until onion is clear.

2. Add remaining ingredients.

3. Cover and boil gently until beans are tender, about 10 minutes.

EGGPLANT-TOMATO COMBO

Four servings, ½ cup each

Per serving:

   Calories: 55
   Total fat: 2.2 grams
   Saturated fat: 0.4 gram
   Cholesterol: 0

---

1 clove garlic, minced
⅓ cup onion, sliced
⅓ cup green pepper strips
2 teaspoons margarine
1 8-ounce can tomatoes
3 cups eggplant, pared, sliced
¼ teaspoon oregano leaves
¼ teaspoon basil leaves
Dash pepper

---

1. Cook garlic, onion, and green pepper in margarine in large frying pan until onion is clear.

2. Break up large pieces of tomato.

3. Add tomatoes, eggplant, and seasonings to onion mixture.

4. Cover and boil gently until vegetables are tender and most of the liquid has evaporated, about 15 minutes. Stir occasionally during cooking.

ORANGE-FLAVORED CARROTS

Four servings, ½ cup each

Per serving:

   Calories: 45
   Total fat: 0.2 gram
   Saturated fat: 0
   Cholesterol: 0

_____

3 cups carrots, sliced

2 tablespoons onion, chopped

1 cup boiling water

⅛ teaspoon salt

2 tablespoons frozen orange juice concentrate

1 teaspoon lemon juice

2 tablespoons vegetable cooking liquid

_____

1. Add carrots and onion to boiling salted water. Cover and boil gently until carrots are tender, about 20 minutes. Drain. Save 2 tablespoons liquid.

2. Add orange juice concentrate, lemon juice, and cooking liquid to drained vegetables. Stir gently. Reheat to serving temperature.

TANGY SPINACH

Four servings, about ⅓ cup each

Per serving:

Calories: 35 with fresh spinach; 45 with frozen spinach
Total fat: 2.4 grams
Saturated fat: 0.4 gram
Cholesterol: 0

_____

1 10-ounce package fresh spinach

2 teaspoons oil

¼ cup onion, chopped

2 tablespoons vinegar

¼ teaspoon salt

¼ teaspoon pepper

_____

1. Wash and trim spinach. Tear into pieces.

2. Cook spinach with water clinging to leaves in covered saucepan until just tender, about 3 minutes. Drain.

3. Heat oil in small frying pan. Add onion and cook, covered, until onion is tender. Stir occasionally.

4. Stir in vinegar and seasonings.

5. Pour hot vinegar mixture over spinach and serve.

Note: Two 10-ounce packages partially thawed, frozen leaf spinach may be used in place of fresh spinach. Servings will be slightly larger.

Salads

VEGETABLE-STUFFED TOMATOES

Four servings, 1 tomato each

Per serving:

    Calories: 65
    Total fat: 0.4 gram
    Saturated fat: trace
    Cholesterol: 0

4 medium tomatoes
½ cup fresh green beans, ½-inch pieces
½ cup frozen whole kernel corn
½ cup boiling water
½ cup zucchini squash, diced
¼ cup celery, thinly sliced
2 green onions, sliced
¼ teaspoon salt
⅓ cup low-calorie dressing (French)
Salad greens as desired

1. Cut a thin slice from top of each tomato. Remove cores. Scoop out as much pulp as possible without breaking tomato shells. Save firm red portion of pulp. Dice and drain.

2. Drain shells. Chill until ready to fill.

3. Add beans and corn to boiling water. Cover and boil gently until beans are tender, about 15 minutes. Drain.

4. Lightly mix cooked vegetables, diced tomato pulp, squash, celery, onions, and salt with dressing.

5. Chill at least 1 hour.

6. Fill chilled tomato shells with vegetable mixture.

7. Serve on crisp salad greens.

Note: For a quick and easy version, use 1½ cups cooked unsalted frozen mixed vegetables in place of corn, beans, and squash.

APPLE-CABBAGE SLAW

Four servings, ½ cup each

Per serving:

    Calories: 35
    Total fat: 0.5 gram
    Saturated fat: 0.2 gram
    Cholesterol: 1 milligram

¼ cup plain low-fat yogurt

¼ teaspoon salt

Dash pepper

2 teaspoons vinegar

¼ teaspoon prepared mustard

1 cup apples, unpared, thinly sliced

2 cups cabbage, shredded

1. Mix yogurt, salt, pepper, vinegar, and mustard thoroughly.
2. Lightly mix apples and cabbage.
3. Pour yogurt mixture over apple-cabbage mixture. Toss lightly.
4. Serve immediately.

JELLIED VEGETABLE SALAD

Four servings, ⅔ cup each
Per serving:
 Calories: 30
 Total fat: 0.1 gram
 Saturated fat: 0
 Cholesterol: 0

---

1 envelope unflavored gelatin
¼ cup water
1½ cups boiling water
2 tablespoons tarragon vinegar
¼ teaspoon salt
½ tablespoon honey
¾ cup cabbage, finely shredded
½ cup carrots, shredded
¼ cup celery, chopped
½ cup cucumber, pared, diced
1 tablespoon green onion, chopped
1 tablespoon pimiento, finely chopped
Salad greens as desired

---

1. Soften gelatin in ¼ cup water for 5 minutes.
2. Add softened gelatin to boiling water. Stir until gelatin is dissolved.

3. Stir in vinegar, salt, and honey.

4. Chill until mixture begins to thicken.

5. Fold in remaining ingredients except salad greens.

6. Pour into a 1-quart mold or 8-inch square pan.

7. Chill until set.

8. Unmold and serve on crisp salad greens.

Breads

BRAN MUFFINS

Eight muffins
Per muffin:
   Calories: 120
   Total fat: 4.5 grams
   Saturated fat: 0.8 gram
   Cholesterol: 35 milligrams

⅔ cup unprocessed whole bran
1 cup whole-wheat flour
2 tablespoons brown sugar, packed
½ tablespoon baking powder
⅛ teaspoon salt
⅔ cup skim milk
1 egg, slightly beaten
2 tablespoons oil

---

1. Preheat oven to 400°F. (hot oven).

2. Grease 8 muffin tins.

3. Mix dry ingredients thoroughly.

4. Mix milk, egg, and oil. Add to dry ingredients. Stir until dry ingredients are barely moistened. Batter will be lumpy.

5. Fill muffin tins two-thirds full.

6. Bake until lightly browned, about 25 minutes.

HERB BREAD

One loaf, 12 slices

Per slice:

  Calories: 95
  Total fat: 3.6 grams
  Saturated fat: 0.6 gram
  Cholesterol: trace

1½ cups whole-wheat flour

2 tablespoons sugar

1 teaspoon baking powder

¼ teaspoon salt

¼ teaspoon ground mace

¼ teaspoon thyme leaves

2 teaspoons caraway seeds

1 egg white, slightly beaten

⅔ cup skim milk

3 tablespoons oil

---

1. Preheat oven to 350°F.

2. Grease 7-by-3-by-2-inch loaf pan lightly with oil.

3. Mix dry ingredients thoroughly.

4. Mix egg white, milk, and oil. Add to dry ingredients. Stir until dry ingredients are barely moistened. Batter will be lumpy.

5. Pour into pan.

6. Bake until batter no longer clings to a toothpick inserted in center, about 55 minutes.

7. Remove from pan. Cool on rack.

WHOLE-WHEAT BREAD

Two loaves, 16 slices each

Per slice:

Calories: 95
Total fat: 2.1 grams
Saturated fat: 0.3 gram
Cholesterol: 0

6 cups whole-wheat flour

1 package active dry yeast (see note below)

1 teaspoon salt

2 cups water

¼ cup oil

2 tablespoons honey

1. Mix 2 cups of the flour with yeast and salt.

2. Heat water and oil together until warm (105° to 115°F.). Add honey. Stir into flour mixture. Beat well.

3. Mix in enough of the remaining flour to make a soft dough that leaves the side of the bowl.

4. Knead on a lightly-floured surface until dough is smooth and elastic, about 15 minutes.

Note: If you use one of the new rapid-rise yeasts, follow the package directions for rising times.

5. Place dough in a greased bowl and turn over once to grease upper side of dough.

6. Cover and let rise in a warm place (80° to 85°F.) until doubled in size, about 1 hour.

7. Grease two 9-by-5-by-3-inch loaf pans.

8. Press dough down to remove air bubbles.

9. Divide dough in half. Shape each half into a loaf. Place in pans.

10. Cover and let rise in a warm place until doubled in size, about 50 minutes.

11. Preheat oven to 375°F.

12. Bake until bread sounds hollow when tapped, about 30 minutes.

13. Remove bread from pans and cool on rack.

Desserts

STEAMED CARROT PUDDING

Eight servings

Per serving:

    Calories: 105
    Total fat: 3.5 grams
    Saturated fat: 0.6 gram
    Cholesterol: 34 milligrams

½ cup whole-wheat flour
¼ teaspoon baking soda
¼ teaspoon baking powder
⅓ cup brown sugar, packed
⅛ teaspoon salt
½ teaspoon ground cinnamon
¼ teaspoon ground nutmeg

1 egg
1 tablespoon margarine, softened
½ cup carrots, grated
½ cup potatoes, grated
¼ teaspoon lemon rind, grated
2 tablespoons walnuts, chopped

---

1. Grease a 2½-cup casserole or small pudding mold.
2. Mix dry ingredients.
3. Beat egg and margarine together. Stir in flour mixture. Mix well.
4. Add remaining ingredients. Mix well.
5. Pour mixture into casserole. Cover tightly with foil.
6. Place casserole on rack in a deep pan with a lid. Add boiling water to come halfway up side of casserole. Casserole should not touch cover of pan.
7. Cover pan and simmer 2 hours.
8. Remove casserole from pan. Cool on rack until lukewarm.
9. Unmold pudding from casserole.
10. Serve warm, or cool completely. To store, wrap in foil and place in refrigerator. For best quality use within 4 or 5 days.

GINGER WHEAT COOKIES

About 5 dozen cookies
Per cookie:
    Calories: 45
    Total fat: 1.9 grams
    Saturated fat: 0.3 gram
    Cholesterol: 0

½ cup oil

½ cup brown sugar, packed

2 egg whites

⅓ cup orange juice

2 cups whole-wheat flour

½ cup unsweetened wheat germ

1 teaspoon baking soda

¼ teaspoon salt

¼ teaspoon ground cloves

2 teaspoons ground ginger

½ cup raisins, chopped

---

1. Preheat oven to 350°F.
2. Mix oil and sugar.
3. Add egg whites and orange juice. Beat until frothy.
4. Mix dry ingredients thoroughly.
5. Add dry ingredients and raisins to oil mixture. Mix well.
6. Drop dough by teaspoons onto ungreased baking sheet, about 2 inches apart.
7. Bake until cookies are lightly browned and feel firm to the touch, about 8 minutes.
8. Remove from baking sheet while still warm.
9. Cool on rack.

WINTER FRUIT CUP

Four servings, about ½ cup each

Per serving:

Calories: 70

Total fat: 0.3 gram

Saturated fat: 0
Cholesterol: 0

½ cup grapes, halved, seeded
½ cup tangerine, sectioned
½ cup apple, unpared, diced
½ cup pear, unpared, diced
½ cup banana, sliced
2 tablespoons frozen orange juice concentrate, thawed

---

1. Mix fruit with orange juice concentrate to coat all pieces.
2. Serve immediately.

IF AT FIRST YOU DON'T SUCCEED . . .

Relapse is a pretty scary word for most ex-smokers. The fear of failing after going through so much effort in giving up cigarettes is a bogeyman which haunts the dreams of many of us who have put out our last cigarette.

The fact remains that many ex-smokers have given in to the temptation to light up at some time, and such a single lapse in willpower does not mean a total defeat or a return to that nasty habit. It is important to remember that. A relapse is not the end of the world! Look at how long you have gone smokeless. Is one slip-up going to stop you from accomplishing what you have set out to do? If at first you don't succeed, try, try again . . .

Sometimes, though, we unwittingly put ourselves in situations where we invite trouble. One example is a situation many of us are familiar with, the high school reunion. It's hard to believe, but there you are after ten years, right back in the old gymnasium. And of course, on this special night, seeing and talking to so many of your old friends, the memories will flow as freely as the drinks. And judging from the number of cigarettes being smoked in the old gym, most of your former classmates are definitely not listening to the surgeon general's advice.

Why is this happy occasion fraught with danger for the new ex-smoker? First of all, the event is probably making you feel a bit anxious. Most of us feel so when we meet with people we knew long ago, but whom we haven't seen for a while. There's also an atmosphere of celebration—drinking and smoking. It's pretty difficult not to get caught up in all this festive spirit. Your guard is also down from the alcohol you've consumed.

This is the perfect relapse situation, according to a new study which statistically examined the reasons why ex-smokers take that first puff again. The statistics were collected from people who called a "Stay Quit Hotline" for help in remaining smokeless.

Ex-smokers were urged to call the hotline from eight A.M. to eleven P.M. daily, whether they had already slipped and taken that first puff or were experiencing a "relapse crisis" in which they were frantically trying to fight the urge. The callers were all counseled and asked a predetermined set of questions.

Two-thirds of the 183 people who called the hotline were women, and 60 percent of the callers had participated in a "quit smoking" program. All the callers had smoked at least ten cigarettes per day and had not smoked for at least two days. The average caller had smoked a little over thirty-four cigarettes per day for almost twenty years, so the study was comprised of some pretty hard-core smokers.

The number of days that the callers had not smoked did, of course, vary, but the average was about ten days—so the group was composed of relatively new ex-smokers. About two out of five users of the service who were interviewed had already relapsed, but most had only smoked one cigarette.

This study gives us some surprising clues as to when, where, and how most former smokers revert to their old habit. The data indicates that such relapse situations are likely to happen at any time of the day, with a slightly greater likelihood during the morning hours. The study also noted that an ex-smoker is more than twice as likely to undergo such a crisis at home as at work or somewhere else such as a restaurant or a friend's home. More than half the time that such a crisis struck, other people, such as family members or co-workers, were present. This was especially true when a relapse situation occurred outside the ex-smoker's home. Interestingly enough, in about half of such situations, one of those others present was smoking.

Of course, this suggests that watching a person smoke can create a powerful urge for a cigarette—not a big secret among us ex-smokers. But multiply this situation by ten—say in that high school gymnasium or a bar—and you have real problems. This is why many "quit smoking" programs strongly advise that new ex-smokers avoid, at least for a while, people who smoke or places like bars that are conducive to smoking.

There are other situations which trigger relapse, the study found, and they involve food and liquids. One-third of the callers to the hotline had suffered their relapse crises either while or shortly after drinking or eating. About 30 percent of the callers said they were eating a meal at the time of their crisis, and about 20 percent were consuming alcohol or coffee.

Now we don't expect you to stop eating, but one suggestion we'd like to reiterate is that you brush your teeth immediately upon completion of your meal. The lingering taste of food in the mouth tends to create a trigger to smoke. The fastest way to douse that desire is to brush your teeth.

Both coffee and alcohol also reinforce the desire to smoke.

Many former smokers have reported that they desired less coffee after they quit smoking, but if you still like the stuff, try to switch to decaffeinated coffee or a cup of tea.

The watchword for ex-smokers who enjoy alcoholic beverages is to have fewer and weaker drinks. If you're drinking beer or wine, try to limit yourself to a glass or two. If you enjoy cocktails, try to dilute them or have the bartender pour you a weak one. And if you're at a party and want to disguise the fact that you're not drinking, try tonic water on the rocks or a Tom Collins mixer on the rocks. Nobody will notice the difference.

As we've previously discussed, emotions can also be a pretty powerful stimulant to light up. The study found that the typical relapse situation took place during a period which 42 percent of the callers described as stressful or anxious. Approximately one-third of those who called were having problems either at work or with their personal relationships.

One-fourth of the hotline's callers reported that they were angry or frustrated, according to the study. This is not surprising, because some research has indicated that nicotine acts to control or diminish anger. Should you be feeling angry or frustrated, review the chapter on breathing exercises. Repeat them as often as necessary.

Depression was also a major complaint to operators of the hotline. At least 22 percent of ex-smokers who phoned reported this emotional state. Of course we now know that depression is a natural reaction to quitting smoking. And, hopefully, you also know that the best way to work yourself through such feelings is by plenty of exercise.

It was not only negative states of mind that callers to the hotline complained of. At least 15 percent of the calls received were from former smokers who said they were experiencing relapse crises while feeling happy or relaxed. When you think about it, being happy is often part of having a good time, which usually includes some socializing. And socializing, as we know, can sometimes subject ex-smokers to some rough tests of willpower and endurance.

Right about now it might be appropriate to talk a bit more about how to handle situations where pressure to smoke might be brought to bear upon you. How, for example, would you respond to a friend who pokes fun at you for not joining him in a smoke? We're going to show you some of what we call "reality survival techniques" to help you make the correct response.

SAY IT AGAIN, SAM

Let's begin by asking a few questions which, as an ex-smoker, you may right now not feel are relevant to your task of surviving pressure situations. But there is a point to these questions, as you soon shall see.

Do you ever feel people take advantage of you? Do you fly off the handle easily? Do you often not trust your own instincts? If you answered yes to any of these questions, you're probably going to need some training in assertiveness if you plan to survive as a nonsmoker.

Assertiveness training operates on the principle that there are basically three types of responses one can make to a negative situation—such as when people are talking loudly in front of you in a movie theater.

An *aggressive* response is one which expresses your feelings, but is done in such a way that you've lost control. This type of response attacks a person rather than their behavior, and creates tension. In such a situation you have not only lost self-control, but some of your self-respect along with it.

A *passive* response is one in which you choose to do nothing. Instead, you take a course of action which allows other people to make choices for you. Your self-respect will probably take another beating in this type of situation, which will only serve to make you feel frustrated and tense.

An *assertive* response not only allows you to express your feelings and stand up for your rights, but it is done in such a manner that it both maintains your self-respect and creates little tension. Such a response is especially important to ex-smokers, because the other two types of reaction create frustration, tension, and lack of self-respect—states of mind that can lead to a desire for a cigarette.

Let's return to our example of people talking loudly in a movie theater. There are three basic ways to handle that situation. The aggressive way would be to say in a loud voice, "Hey, why don't you shut up? Do you think you own the theater or something?" The passive reaction, of course, would be simply to say nothing and suffer through the situation. The assertive approach would be to tell the noisemakers in a normal tone of voice, "I realize that you're really enjoying this movie and that's why you're talking. But the rest of us can't hear. So please be quiet."

Even if the people still refuse to quiet down, you've stated your feelings in a nonthreatening way. You've maintained your self-respect by speaking up as well. Maintaining such self-respect is extremely important to us new nonsmokers, because it means we'll be more likely to listen to ourselves when it comes to resisting an urge to smoke or eat.

Let's take another example. Say you're at lunch with a friend who asks to borrow twenty-five dollars, and you know you can't afford to spare the money. What are your options?

The aggressive response would be to say in an angry manner, "Listen, I'm sick and tired of this. What do you think I am, a bank? We make about the same amount of money, but I manage mine." The passive reaction would be to say, "Oh, sure," and take out your checkbook while you're hurting all the time. The assertive approach would be to say something like, "You'll have to ask someone else. I really can't spare the money."

Now let's look at a situation that we're likely to encounter as new ex-smokers who are concerned about our weight. You're at your mother's house for dinner and she's surprised you by baking your favorite pie. You've told her several times that you can't eat pie because you're on a diet, but she just won't take no for an answer. How would you handle the situation?

The aggressive approach would be to say in an angry tone of voice, "Look, how many times do I have to tell you that I'm on a diet. You're driving me crazy." This only causes a lot of hurt. The passive response would be to say, "Well, I guess one piece wouldn't hurt me." You are literally going to swallow your self-respect. The assertive, and perhaps the best, approach would be to say politely, "I'm sorry, mom, but I really have to watch my weight since I quit smoking. The pie looks delicious and I wish I could have some, but taking one piece of pie is just like smoking one cigarette."

Here is one of the toughest social situations you may have to handle as a new nonsmoker. You are at a party and an old friend comes up to talk to you. He lights up, sees that you aren't, and says, "Hey, buddy, are you out of smokes?" So he offers you one. You then tell him about your decision to quit smoking and he gives you one of those looks. "Oh, no," he says, "don't tell me you've become one of those health freaks. They really drive me up the wall." The social pressure is really on now. How should you respond?

The aggressive response would elicit an angry reaction.

"Don't jump on me just because you obviously can't quit," you would shout. "Talk about freaks . . . look at you, you're a human chimney." The passive reaction would have you making some lame excuse, such as "I'm under doctor's orders not to smoke." The assertive response would be to say, "If taking care of my health makes me some kind of freak, well, then, I guess I am."

Amazingly enough, in those first crucial months of not smoking, the person you might have to be most assertive with is yourself! Sometimes, to drag out an old expression, we really can be our own worst enemy. This is an example how:

Say you're at a meeting and are about to deliver a speech. You're understandably nervous, and a little voice inside you keeps saying, "You've got to calm down or you're really going to mess up out there." That same little voice continues, "I've got to have just one cigarette. It'll calm me down and get me through this speech."

Now you are in conflict with yourself. It is a perfect opportunity to put a little of that assertiveness training to work on your behalf. Your assertive response should go something like this: "I'm going to feel so good about myself after I've made this speech without a cigarette. This will really be a milestone. I know I can do it without that cigarette."

As with any new technique, practice makes perfect. Why not make up some of your own reality survival situations and think about what your assertive response would be. Practice in front of a mirror and speak your responses aloud. Try these tips for your delivery: Make eye contact. Look straight at the person to whom you're talking. Stand straight. The way you stand often influences the way you feel about yourself, and often you are judged by your posture. Speak with conviction. You have a right to. Look at all you've accomplished in such a short time . . .

F·O·U·R·T·E·E·N

VISUALIZATION:
TO BE OR NOT TO BE

We've seen that assertive behavior is not only a good technique to utilize during those first crucial months of not smoking, but in all areas of your life as well.

Now let's examine another technique that will help you cope with your new smoke-free lifestyle—visualization. Some of you may only be vaguely familiar with the term, while others may not have ever heard of this concept.

Actually, the term is a fancy way to describe a pretty simple technique. The playwright, William Shakespeare, was familiar with visualization when he wrote, "Assume a virtue if you have it not." It is a principle that has been adopted by thousands of people throughout history.

What it all boils down to is that visualization means utilizing the powers of your imagination to attain whatever goals you set for yourself. Visualize your goals and they will come true. If you want money, success, or a new car, create a mental picture of what you want and hold that thought in your mind.

As a new ex-smoker, visualization is an important technique for you to practice and become familiar with. It is simply not enough to feel great that you have finally stopped smoking. You must take the process one step further—actually see, or visualize, yourself as a successful ex-smoker in the years to come. In Shakespeare's own words, "assume" your success.

Let's take a simple, everyday example. Two cooks are going to bake a cake. They're making the same identical cake—using identical ingredients and methods. Yet one cook's cake turns out dry, partially burnt—let's say it's just barely edible. The second cook's cake is moist, flaky, and perfectly baked. How is this possible?

Now let's retreat a bit and look at the actual baking session. Cook number one began baking with a pretty good case of the jitters. She is nervous because other cakes she's baked have failed. Believe it or not, she is now transferring these apprehensions to the cake she is baking. Cook number two, meanwhile, begins her baking with a picture in mind of the mouth-watering creation that is going to emerge from her oven. She knows that cake is going to be great and, guess what? It is.

There are subconscious forces afoot whether we choose to believe in them or not. It was a scientist of no minor stature—the great Sigmund Freud himself—who first pointed out the powerful force within us which he called the subconscious mind. Unlike the conscious mind, the subconscious never sleeps. This force is constantly at work shaping our thoughts, feelings, and actions. A person with a clear goal in mind will plant that image in his subconscious mind. He will bring those subconscious powers into play by creating mental pictures of what he wants to accomplish. And more likely than not he will succeed at what he wants to do.

Okay, let's bring this idea back home. Here we are as an

ex-smoker who has just been invited to a dinner party. It's your first test of willpower. How will I ever make it through the evening without a cigarette, you wonder. As the hour approaches, your anxiety level begins to peak. You watch the minutes tick by with a sense of gloom. You're feeling exhausted and you haven't even dressed for the party yet. Is there anything you can do to ease all this anxiety and worry? Certainly there is. The answer lies in doing a visualization exercise—preparing yourself mentally for a good time this evening, and without cigarettes—rather than filling your head with negative thoughts and doubts.

You probably remember from high school science that two objects cannot fill the same space at the same time. Well, think of your mind in exactly those terms. Your mind cannot be filled with negative thoughts and doubts if you've already filled it with positive ones. So let the positive thoughts flow! Visualize!

How *exactly* does one do visualization? There are many ways, all of them similar and all of them simple to do. We have our own favorite which we'd be more than glad to share with you.

Begin as you would if you were practicing the meditation technique described earlier in this book. Find a quiet place, disconnect the telephone, sit comfortably on a straight-backed chair or on the floor, and place your hands on your thighs palms up. Ten minutes of time is all that will be required of you, although with practice you may want to spend twenty minutes or more each day visualizing whatever goals or desires you have in mind. For the moment, however, let's concentrate on that approaching dinner party instead of visualizing a new job or a check in the mail.

It is always a good idea to begin your visualization exercise by imagining a ball of white light hovering just above and in front of your head. Let this ball of white light shoot its rays into your head and through your body. Imagine the light filling your neck, chest, arms, legs—every cell in the body. You are bathed in this white light—protected by it. This light protects you from any would-be negative influences that might be afloat in the world.

Now you're ready to begin the second phase of your visualization. Imagine yourself beautifully dressed or handsomely attired and knocking on the door of the house where the dinner party is being held. You are feeling calm, confident, and relaxed. You are radiating the healthful energy of someone who has quit smoking and knows that he or she is looking better and feeling better.

Visualize the conversation between your host and yourself. The compliments on your looks, your wardrobe, and how calm you feel without any cigarette as a crutch. Oh, yes. You're going to have a wonderful time tonight. It was foolish to have felt so anxious.

Continue your visualization. Imagine the delicious meal, the delightful dinner conversation, the smooth after-dinner drinks, and the charming guests. You are not nervous, not tense—see yourself as you would like to be at that party—and, most important of all, you feel no need to fish for a cigarette. The party is a success and so are you. Visualize yourself getting ready to go home and almost sorry that this wonderful time is ending.

When you have visualized the entire dinner party—especially your successful role in it—it is time to open your eyes. Do so slowly, take your time. Relax. Feel confident. What you have visualized is almost certain to come true. Keep that mental imagery in mind as you dress for the party. If, just before you leave, you need to run it through one more time, take another five or ten minutes and do so. Now go and enjoy yourself!

Visualization is a wonderful mental technique that can

be applied to all aspects of your life. There are several books available on the subject and they're worth the cover price. Remember, all you have to do is picture yourself as a successful nonsmoker, and you will be just that . . .

ONE IS THE
LONELIEST NUMBER

To survive as an ex-smoker, it may be important for you to link up with a support group, if one exists, or, if not, to consider starting one of your own.

Everybody needs a little help sometimes—especially if you've put out that last cigarette and are experiencing any kind of stress or anxiety. Coping by yourself with such feelings is often a difficult task, which is why we suggested earlier in the book that you involve relatives and friends in your efforts to remain smokeless.

But let's face it: when it comes down to it, nobody but another ex-smoker will really understand what you are going through. Which is why there is a need for ex-smokers to band together for positive reinforcement and to share common experiences, problems, and solutions. There is a special bond among people who share the same experiences; it begins when one person says to another, "I know just how you feel."

The mutual-help movement has grown rapidly in this country over the last decade or so. Millions of people whose problems and needs are not being met through formal health care, social services, or counseling programs are finding alternatives to coping alone in self-help groups. Among the estimated half million mutual-help groups in existence, there are groups to deal with almost every human problem; but each of them has the same underlying purpose: to provide emotional support and practical help in dealing with a problem common to all its members.

The structure of mutual-help groups and the way they serve their members depends primarily on their goals. Each local group determines its own programs and meeting schedules. Typically, groups hold regular meetings in church halls, public buildings, or other no-rent or low-rent facilities. Many small groups meet in a member's home.

Programs for those meetings can include group discussions, study groups, visiting speakers, and other activities that inform members and help them to build confidence. To supplement the personal support gained from meetings, the group may offer additional services or even start a newsletter. Since the groups are run by members for members, there are seldom any professional salaries or overhead costs. Many groups are entirely self-supporting through members' voluntary contributions or minimal dues.

What happens at such meetings? The process begins with a first gathering. It is at this meeting that members are made aware of how hard it is to deal with problems alone. Everyone then shares common problems, experiences, and solutions. Goals—both short-range and long-range—are often set. Everyone is given the freedom to draw on the strength of the group as needed and to extend strength to others when possible. In general, there is an atmosphere of acceptance that encourages members to share their fears, frustrations, and successes. From there, they can begin to communicate more openly, view their problems more objectively, and find more effective coping strategies.

You may already have heard about a mutual-help group that deals with your concerns. There are a number of ways to get more information. Some of the larger groups are listed by subject in the phone directory, and the names and phone numbers of many more are available from hospitals and local health and social-service agencies. If you're interested in a group that does not have a unit in your area, its central office will provide information on how to organize one.

One good source is the public library. Directories of self-help groups are generally available there. Comprehensive information and assistance—including how to organize a group—can be obtained by writing or calling the National Self-Help Clearinghouse at the address below.

Frank Riessman, PhD, Director
National Self-Help Clearinghouse
City University of New York Graduate Center, Room 1206A
33 West Forty-second Street
New York, New York 10036
212-840-1259

The National Self-Help Clearinghouse operates units throughout the country, and we have included a list of such centers at the end of this chapter.

You may want to start a self-help group of your own— one which deals exclusively with the problems faced by new ex-smokers. Your first problem in getting a group started is to locate at least one other person sharing your concern. This could be done by contacting a hospital or any agency—such as the heart association in your area—which operates "quit smoking" programs.

Once you've located a group of interested individuals,

schedule an informal meeting. This could be in your home or in a local public facility.

The group's first task is to decide the purpose of the group. Keep it as general as possible. This general purpose can include a number of goals which the group can decide upon as it progresses.

There are some early decisions a new group faces. First is a meeting space. Meeting in a member's home is not always the best solution even for a small group. Pressure is put on the host which may interfere with his or her ability to grow in the group. Look for an outside space. It may have to be paid for by passing the hat.

The group must also decide on structure. Keep it simple! Don't take on more structure than you need. A small group does not need a board of directors, but may need a member to act as facilitator of the discussion. Base your decision on what will best serve the group's purpose.

Who is in and who is out as a member? Decide for yourselves who can be part of your group. Will it be just ex-smokers, or their friends and relatives as well?

Grab all the free publicity you can in community newspapers, television, and radio. Put up flyers in strategic locations; get the word out. The most effective way to build a membership (and to keep it) is to start people chains. People need to be engaged on a one-to-one basis. In turn, they need to be encouraged to bring in other people.

You may want to involve some professionals to help get your group going. As long as the members themselves take responsibility for the group and don't become dependent on a professional, this relationship can work for the good.

Don't amass more money than you need. Big balances are for corporations. Self-help groups can often survive on free-will donations from participants. When more funds are needed for a particular special purpose they can be raised as required.

Sharing is the key to effectiveness. When you hear another person's story, you feel less alone. When you share your own story, it becomes less scary. How this sharing can be done will depend upon the size of your group. Most group discussions can't include more than ten people if all members are to participate fully. If you have a larger group, don't neglect the opportunity to break down into small groups for discussion.

Plan to have something for people to do when they come to the group. If people can't participate themselves and get a sense of self-worth through contributing to the group, then they won't stay for long.

Directory of Self-Help Groups

California

Carol Eisman, Public Education Specialist
California Self-Help Resource Center
UCLA, 2349 Franz Hall
405 Hilgard Avenue
Los Angeles, California 90024
213-825-3522

Geri Stewart, Coordinator
Self-Help Clearinghouse of Merced County
Mental Health Association of Merced County
PO Box 343
Merced, California 95341
209-723-8861

Self-Help Network & Clearinghouse/Santa Maria
Mental Health Association of Santa Maria
PO Box 104
Santa Maria, California 93456
805-922-2165

Ruth Tebbets, Director
Bay Area Self-Help Clearinghouse
San Francisco Mental Health Association
2398 Pine Street
San Francisco, California 94115
415-921-4401

Janet Manfred, Coordinator
Sacramento Self-Help
Mental Health Association of Sacramento
5370 Elvas Avenue
Sacramento, California 95819
916-456-2070

Ellen Murphey, Executive Director
San Diego Self-Help Clearinghouse
PO Box 86246
San Diego, California 92138
619-275-2344

Connecticut

Vicki Spiro Smith, Coordinator
Connecticut SH/Mutual Support Network
Consultation Center
19 Howe Street
New Haven, Connecticut 06511
203-789-7645

Illinois

Leonard D. Borman, PhD, Director
Self-Help Center
1600 Dodge Avenue, Suite S-122
Evanston, Illinois 60201
312-328-0470

Kansas

Evelyn Middelstadt, MSW, Coordinator
Sedgwick County Self-Help Center
PO Box 8511
Wichita, Kansas 67208
316-686-1205

Michigan

Rob Hess and Charles Livingston, Coordinators
Barrien County Self-Help Clearinghouse
Riverwood Community Mental Health Center
2681 Morton Avenue
St. Joseph, Michigan 49085
616-983-7781

Minnesota

Gloria Johnson, Information Specialist
Mutual Help Resource Center
Wilder Foundation Community Care Unit
919 Lafond Avenue
St. Paul, Minnesota 55104
612-642-4060

Nebraska

Barbara Fox, Director
Self-Help Information Services
1601 Euclid Avenue
Lincoln, Nebraska 68502
402-476-9668

New Jersey

Edward J. Madera, Director
New Jersey Self-Help Clearinghouse
CMHC
St. Clare's Hospital
Denville, New Jersey 07834
201-625-7101

New York

Frances J. Dory, Director
New York City Self-Help Clearinghouse
186 Joralemon Street
Brooklyn, New York 11201
718-852-4290

Carol Berkvist, CSS Coordinator
Brooklyn Self-Help Clearinghouse
Heights/Hill MHS
50 Court Street
Brooklyn, New York 11201
718-834-7341

Audrey Lief, Coordinator
Long Island Self-Help Clearinghouse
Commack College Center
6350 Jericho Turnpike
Commack, New York 11725
516-499-8800 x501

Leslie Borck, Director
Westchester Self-Help Clearinghouse
Westchester Community College
75 Grasslands Road
Valhalla, New York 10595
914-347-3620

Fred Meservey, Coordinator
NY State Self-Help Clearinghouse
Council on Children and Families
Empire State Plaza Tower 2
Albany, New York 12224
518-474-6682

Self-Help Clearinghouse Director
Regional Self-Help Clearinghouse/Lockport
Mental Health Association of Niagara County
88 East Avenue
Lockport, New York 14094
716-433-3780

Self-Help Clearinghouse Director
Regional Self-Help Clearinghouse/Rochester
Mental Health Chapter of Rochester/Monroe
973 East Avenue
Rochester, New York 14607
716-271-3540

Self-Help Clearinghouse Director
Regional Self-Help Clearinghouse/Syracuse
The Volunteer Center
115 East Jefferson Street, Suite 300
Syracuse, New York 13202
315-474-7011

Self-Help Clearinghouse Director
Regional Self-Help Clearinghouse/Schenectady
Human Services Planning Council of Schenectady, Inc.
432 State Street
Schenectady, New York 12305
518-372-3395

Self-Help Clearinghouse Director
Regional Self-Help Clearinghouse/Elmira
Economic Opportunity Program, Inc.
318 Madison Avenue
Elmira, New York 14901

Self-Help Clearinghouse Director
Regional Self-Help Clearinghouse/Potsdam
Reachout of St. Lawrence County, Inc.
203 Sisson Hall
Potsdam College
Potsdam, New York 13676

Self-Help Clearinghouse Director
Regional Self-Help Clearinghouse/Amsterdam
St. Mary's Hospital
427 Guy Park Avenue
Amsterdam, New York 12010

Self-Help Clearinghouse Director
Dutchess County Self-Help Clearinghouse
United Way of Dutchess County
PO Box 832
75 Market Street
Poughkeepsie, New York 12601

Oregon

Nancy Barron, Director
Portland Self-Help Information Service
718 Burnside Avenue, 5th floor
Portland, Oregon 97209
503-229-4040

Pennsylvania

Jared Hermalin, Director
Philadelphia Self-Help Clearinghouse
John F. Kennedy CMHC
112 North Broad Street, 6th floor
Philadelphia, Pennsylvania 19102
215-568-0860 x266

Arlene Hopkins, Executive Director
Self-Help Information and Networking Exchange
Voluntary Action Center of Northeast Pennsylvania
200 Adams Street
Scranton, Pennsylvania 18503
717-961-1234

Betty Hepner, Coordinator
Self-Help Group Network
c/o 2839 Beechwood Boulevard
Pittsburgh, Pennsylvania 15216
412-521-9822

Texas

Carol Madison, Staff Associate
Mental Health Association of Dallas County
2500 Maple Avenue
Dallas, Texas 75201-1998
214-871-2420

Steve Summers, Program Specialist
Tarrant County Self-Help Clearinghouse
MHA of Tarrant County
3136 West 4th Street
Fort Worth, Texas 76107-2113
817-335-5405

Vermont

Joanne Brooking, Coordinator
Vermont Self-Help Clearinghouse
c/o Parents Anonymous
PO Box 829
Montpelier, Vermont 05602
802-229-5724; 800-544-5030

Virginia

Linda Figueroa, Coordinator
Greater Washington Self-Help Coalition
MHA of Northern Virginia
100 North Washington Street, Suite 232
Falls Church, Virginia 22046
703-536-4100

Wisconsin

Deborah Mosley, President
Mutual Aid Self-Help Association
MASHA
PO Box 09304
Milwaukee, Wisconsin 53209
414-461-1466

SURVIVAL QUIZZES

Now that you've finished reading this book, we're going to put some of what you have learned to the test. In the following pages we are going to test your knowledge in such areas as controlling and breaking smoking habits, assertiveness, exercise, and diet. All the quizzes have been formulated by the US Department of Health and Human Services Public Health Service.

Quiz 1: Controlling Smoking Habits

This quiz consists of 20 statements about controlling smoking habits. Some of the statements are true and some are false. Put your answer in "True or False" column.

	True or False
1. Meditation is an effective way to try to keep from smoking when you feel the need to relax.	_____
2. Eating something is an effective way to try to keep from smoking when you are tense and angry.	_____
3. When you are trying to stop smoking, the number of things that make you want to smoke will usually decrease.	_____
4. Understanding why you smoke means being aware of the situations, times and places that make you want to smoke.	_____
5. Different things make different people want to smoke.	_____
6. Rewarding yourself for not smoking usually is of little help in stopping smoking.	_____
7. Eating something is an effective way to try to keep from smoking when you feel the need to be stimulated.	_____
8. A particular technique for avoiding smoking usually will work effectively for all smokers.	_____
9. Brisk walking is an effective way to try to keep from smoking when you feel the need to be stimulated.	_____
10. Drawing is an effective way to try to keep from smoking when you feel the need to do something with your hands.	_____
11. Changing routine activities is an effective way to try to keep from smoking when you feel the need to relax.	_____
12. Techniques for avoiding smoking need to be practiced in order to be used effectively.	_____
13. Certain times or places that are part of a person's daily routine can make that person want to smoke.	_____
14. Smoking is a habit that occurs only when an individual thinks about it.	_____

	True or False
15. Drinking nonalcoholic beverages is an effective way to keep from smoking when you feel tense.	————
16. Reading is an effective way to try to keep from smoking when you feel bored.	————
17. To be effective, techniques for avoiding smoking should satisfy a person's desire to smoke.	————
18. A technique for avoiding smoking will be most effective if it is an activity commonly associated with smoking.	————
19. Eating sugarless candy is an effective way to try to keep from smoking when you feel the need for oral gratification.	————
20. Doing deep breathing exercises is an effective way to keep from smoking when you feel the need to do something with your hands.	————

Answers

1. T	**11.** F
2. F	**12.** T
3. F	**13.** T
4. T	**14.** F
5. T	**15.** F
6. F	**16.** T
7. F	**17.** T
8. F	**18.** F
9. T	**19.** T
10. T	**20.** F

Quiz 2: Breaking Smoking Habits

This quiz presents descriptions of people who want to break their smoking habits. Read each description and select from the four choices the most healthy and effective way to handle each situation. Circle the letter preceding your choice.

1. Angela usually smokes while she is drinking a cup of coffee with breakfast. The most healthy and effective way to handle this particular smoking trigger would be to:

   a. take several deep breaths before starting to eat.

   b. stay at the table for a few minutes after breakfast.

   c. drink a beverage other than coffee with breakfast.

   d. skip breakfast and have a cup of coffee later.

2. At least once a day, Danny smokes a cigarette because it tastes so good. The most healthy and effective way to handle this particular smoking situation would be to:

   a. have something like raw vegetables or a piece of gum available to chew.

   b. sit quietly for a few minutes whenever the urge to smoke occurs.

   c. wait for half an hour after first wanting the cigarette before smoking it.

   d. have something like a pencil or some paper clips available to handle.

3. Rhonda likes to smoke when she is out with friends. The most healthy and effective way to handle this particular smoking situation would be to:

   a. take part in some physical activities.

   b. get together with her friends in places where smoking is not allowed.

   c. carry only a few cigarettes when getting together with friends.

   d. meet her friends a half hour later than usual for several weeks.

4. One of the reasons Raymond smokes is because of the pleasure he gets from lighting a cigarette and watching the smoke rise. The most healthy and effective way to handle this particular smoking trigger would be to:

a. switch the brand of cigarettes he is smoking for a while.

b. have some fruit juice or soda water to drink.

c. rearrange the furniture in the rooms where he usually smokes.

d. work on a hobby that requires use of the eyes and hands.

5. Sandy frequently smokes a cigarette at the end of a meal. The most healthy and effective way to handle this trigger would be to:

a. read a book or magazine during the meal.

b. leave the table immediately after eating and start another activity.

c. take several deep breaths throughout the meal.

d. have an extra dessert as a reward for not smoking.

6. Pamela frequently smokes when she is feeling tense or anxious. The most healthy and effective way to handle this particular smoking trigger would be to:

a. learn a relaxation routine such as deep breathing.

b. spend as much time as possible in places where smoking is not allowed.

c. ease her tension by smoking only half a cigarette.

d. tackle tension-producing activities at different times of the day.

7. Kevin smokes cigarettes to help him wake up in the morning. The most healthy and effective way to handle this particular smoking trigger would be to:

a. put his alarm clock across the room so he must get out of bed to turn it off.

b. wait until after breakfast to have his first cigarette.

c. do some physical exercise such as stretching or deep breathing when he gets up.

d. sleep with the windows open so his bedroom is cool when he wakes up.

8. Mark smokes to maintain his energy level during the day. The most healthy and effective way to handle this particular smoking cue would be to:

   a. take a few minutes to stretch or jog in place.

   b. drink soft drinks or eat candy.

   c. picture himself as a nonsmoker.

   d. plan his day so that tiring tasks are scheduled in the morning.

9. At the end of a day, Maria smokes a cigarette to help her relax. The most healthy and effective way to handle this particular smoking cue would be to:

   a. change to a brand of cigarettes that is not as tasty.

   b. eat a low-calorie bedtime snack.

   c. take a warm bath or shower.

   d. learn to do an activity such as drawing or painting.

Answers

1. *c*	**6.** *a*
2. *a*	**7.** *c*
3. *b*	**8.** *a*
4. *d*	**9.** *c*
5. *b*	

Quiz 3: Smoking and Assertiveness

This test presents descriptions of people who feel uncomfortable because others are smoking or asking them to smoke, a situation which you, as a new ex-smoker, may soon find yourself in. Select among the possible options a course of action that incorporates the assertiveness techniques discussed in Chapter 13, "Say It Again, Sam." Circle the appropriate answer.

1. Carol is watching television with her husband and he is smoking. Carol has been trying to stop smoking, but the smell of her husband's cigarette smoke is weakening her willpower. To act assertively, Carol should:

   a. ask her husband if he would smoke fewer cigarettes while they are together.

   b. ask her husband if he would smoke in another room.

   c. move to where she can sit near an open window and breathe fresh air rather than cigarette smoke.

   d. none of the above.

2. George and Susan are spending an evening together. After dinner, Susan suggests that they relax by the fire with after-dinner drinks and cigarettes. To act assertively, George should:

   a. tell Susan he doesn't want to smoke.

   b. tell Susan that he has a better idea and ask her to go for a walk.

   c. hold a lighted cigarette without actually smoking it.

   d. none of the above.

3. Ann has recently stopped smoking, but she finds it hard to control her desire to smoke at the end of a meal. She is at lunch with Bob, a good friend, who prepares to light a cigarette as soon as their plates are cleared from the table. To act assertively, Ann should:

   a. tell the waiter that it's hard for her to resist smoking when someone else is smoking.

   b. ask Bob to please wait to smoke until she has left.

   c. order a dessert to help her ignore Bob's smoking.

   d. none of the above.

4. When Alan decided to quit smoking, he searched his possessions and threw away all the cigarettes he found. His wife Paula still smokes, and she leaves her cigarettes scattered all over the house. To act assertively, Alan should:

   a. ask Paula if she would keep her cigarettes someplace where he can't find them.

   b. throw away any of Paula's cigarettes that he finds lying around.

    c. ask Paula if she would smoke only cigarette brands that he does not particularly enjoy.

    d. none of the above.

5. While John and several of his friends are watching a football game on television, a pack of cigarettes is passed around. When everyone except John takes a cigarette, one friend wonders aloud if John is ever going to grow up. To act assertively, John should:

    a. take a cigarette but not light it.

    b. tell his friends to put out their cigarettes because they are dumb to smoke.

    c. ignore the comment and concentrate on the football game.

    d. none of the above.

6. While at a party, Mark is talking with Ruth, an old friend. Ruth knows that Mark is trying to stop smoking, so she decides to offer Mark a cigarette to test his willpower. To act assertively, Mark should:

    a. tell Ruth that she has much less willpower than he does.

    b. accept the cigarette, saying that he will smoke it later.

    c. inform Ruth that he no longer smokes.

    d. none of the above.

7. Nancy is on a date with Tom. To impress her, Tom lights two cigarettes and offers Nancy one, saying that she will look sexy if she smokes a cigarette. To act assertively, Nancy should:

    a. change the subject by asking Tom whether he thinks her new hairdo is attractive.

    b. take the cigarette he offers, then hold it in her hand without smoking it for a few minutes.

    c. turn down the offer, saying she doesn't enjoy smoking.

    d. none of the above.

8. David is waiting to see his lawyer. Another man who is seated in the waiting room is smoking one cigarette after another, and the smoke is beginning to irritate David's eyes. To act assertively, David should:

a. close his eyes to reduce the amount of irritation from the smoke.

b. tell the man that the smoke is irritating his eyes and ask if he would stop smoking or go outside.

c. complain to the receptionist about how smoky the waiting room is getting, using a voice loud enough for the smoker to hear.

d. none of the above.

9. Louise is standing in line at the market, waiting to check out. The woman behind her lights a cigarette and the smoke blows into Louise's face. To act assertively, Louise should:

a. tell the woman that she is inconsiderate.

b. ask the woman if she would blow the smoke in the other direction.

c. move to another checkout line.

d. none of the above.

10. Michael, who does not smoke, pretended to smoke a cigarette as part of his role in a play. Afterward, his girlfriend Jane tells him that smoking made him look more attractive. She asks him to have a cigarette at a party. To act assertively, Michael should:

a. tell Jane that he doesn't want to smoke in order to create an "image."

b. accept the cigarette and hold it but refrain from actually smoking it.

c. pretend that he didn't hear her and ask Jane if she would like to dance.

d. none of the above.

Answers

1. *b*	**6.** *c*
2. *a*	**7.** *c*
3. *b*	**8.** *b*
4. *a*	**9.** *d*
5. *d*	**10.** *a*

Quiz 4: Responding to Others about Smoking

Now that you yourself are a nonsmoker, people will look to you for guidance. The following statements either express a person's feelings about his or her efforts to stop smoking, or request assistance from you in that person's effort to give up cigarettes. You are to choose from among four statements the one response that best communicates acceptance and understanding of the fictitious person's situation.

1. *Dan* says: "I'm trying not to smoke, but I feel left out when I'm with my friends and they are all smoking." The response that best communicates acceptance and understanding of Dan's situation is:

    a. "You should probably find a new group of friends who are non-smokers.

    b. "There's no reason to feel left out just because you're not smoking and others are."

    c. "You feel left out when people around you are smoking and you are not."

    d. "You smoke in order to be accepted by others."

2. *Doris* says: "I'm pleasantly surprised to find I can still enjoy a cup of coffee even if I'm not smoking a cigarette." The response that best communicates acceptance and understanding of Doris's situation is:

    a. "It was foolish of you to assume that your enjoyment of coffee depended on smoking a cigarette."

    b. "You're pleased to find out that quitting smoking hasn't changed your enjoyment of coffee."

    c. "The next thing you should try is going without an after-dinner cigarette."

    d. "Smoking is still bad for you unless you give it up completely."

3. *Patrick* says: "I feel like I can't start the day if I don't have my morning cigarette." The response that best communicates acceptance and understanding of Patrick's situation is:

    a. "You know you don't need a cigarette to start your day."

    b. "You should get out of bed and run around the block to wake up in the morning."

    c. "If you give in to your urge to smoke in the morning, you'll be right back where you started."

    d. "You find it difficult to start the day when you go without smoking a cigarette."

4. *Janet* says: "I get nervous and feel as if I need something to do when I'm at a party now that I don't smoke." The response that best communicates acceptance and understanding of Janet's situation is:

    a. "You get nervous at social gatherings since you quit smoking."

    b. "You used to use smoking as a crutch and hide your nervousness behind a cigarette."

    c. "Try eating something to keep your mind off of smoking."

    d. "You never should have smoked at parties in the first place."

5. *Kenneth* says: "I used to think that smoking during my work breaks helped me relax, but now that I've quit smoking I go back to work even more relaxed." The response that best communicates acceptance and understanding of Kenneth's situation is:

    a. "The next thing you should do is try to stop smoking at home."

    b. "The problem was that you jumped to the conclusion that smoking helped you to relax."

    c. "It's ridiculous to think that smoking can help a person relax."

    d. "You've found out that by giving up smoking at work you've made your breaks even more relaxing."

6. *Paula* says: "I would like to spend the evening at home tonight because if we go out with our friends who smoke, I'll want to smoke too." The response that best communicates acceptance and understanding of Paula's situation is:

    a. "You don't have enough willpower around people who smoke."

b. "You feel that around smokers, you'll get an urge to smoke, so tonight you'd rather we stayed home."

c. "There's no reason for you to smoke, even if your friends are smoking."

d. "You'll be sorry if you let our friends tempt you to start smoking again."

7. *Robert* says: "Whenever I see Jim's cigarettes lying around the apartment, I'm tempted to smoke one." The response that best communicates acceptance and understanding of Robert's situation is:

a. "You are tempted to smoke when you see cigarettes."

b. "Go to a different room when you see cigarettes lying around."

c. "Think about how dangerous smoking is whenever you feel the urge to smoke."

d. "You can't be serious about quitting if you're tempted to smoke every time you see a cigarette package."

8. *Alan* says: "You could be very helpful by refusing to give me a cigarette tonight at the party, even if I ask you for one." The response that best communicates acceptance and understanding of Alan's situation is:

a. "You don't need my help to keep you from smoking tonight."

b. "Stay away from all the smokers at the party tonight."

c. "You'll be sorry if you just rely on me to keep you from smoking."

d. "You want me to help you tonight by turning down your requests for cigarettes."

9. *Gwen* says: "When Sue lights a cigarette, the smell of the smoke makes me want a cigarette." The response that best communicates acceptance and understanding of Gwen's situation is:

a. "If you give in even once, it will be harder to resist the next time."

b. "When you smell the smoke, just tell yourself that cigarettes don't taste as good as they smell."

c. "You feel as if you would like a cigarette when you smell her cigarette smoke."

d. "There's no reason for you to want a cigarette just because she's having one."

10. *Marcia* says: "Whenever I go to lunch with my friends, I have a hard time not smoking because they all smoke." The response that best communicates acceptance and understanding of Marcia's situation is:

    a. "Go to lunch with nonsmokers."

    b. "You find it hard to avoid smoking when your friends smoke at lunch."

    c. "You should try not to go to lunch with those friends."

    d. "You must need approval from your friends if you need to smoke when they do."

11. *Tom* says: "I've been happier since I started taking walks after dinner instead of smoking." The response that best communicates acceptance and understanding of Tom's situation is:

    a. "You feel better since you've replaced cigarette smoking after dinner with walking."

    b. "You're happier because walking is good exercise."

    c. "It's good that you've stopped smoking after dinner because smoking can cause cancer."

    d. "Find someone to walk with you because it will be more fun that way."

12. *Robin* says: "I'm having a hard time quitting smoking because the only way I can relax is to smoke a cigarette." The response that best communicates acceptance and understanding of Robin's situation is:

    a. "Smoking in order to relax is a bad habit."

    b. "You don't understand what relaxation is."

    c. "Don't let yourself smoke when you're upset."

    d. "It's tough for you to give up smoking because you feel you need to smoke in order to relax."

13. *Michael* says: "I feel great about myself because I didn't smoke a single cigarette when we were playing golf today." The response that best communicates acceptance and understanding of Michael's situation is:

    a. "You should have had the sense to quit long ago."

b. "The main reason you have been smoking is because your friends smoke."

c. "You're pleased because you were able to avoid smoking while playing golf."

d. "I hope you never smoke again because it is so bad for your health."

14. *Mary* says: "I'm pleasantly surprised that I was able to go to a party and not smoke a single cigarette." The response that best communicates acceptance and understanding of Mary's situation is:

a. "You're pleased that you were able to avoid smoking at a party."

b. "You're happy because you finally gave up your bad habit."

c. "You used to smoke at parties because of the social pressure you felt."

d. "Keep it up and don't ever smoke at a party again."

15. *Jim* says: "I'm angry because the people in my car pool smoke even though I've asked them not to." The response that best communicates acceptance and understanding of Jim's situation is:

a. "The people that you ride with must be very inconsiderate."

b. "You're upset because the people in your car pool continue to smoke even though you asked them not to."

c. "Ask them again not to smoke."

d. "You probably didn't ask them in the right way."

Answers

1. *c*	**9.** *c*
2. *b*	**10.** *b*
3. *d*	**11.** *a*
4. *a*	**12.** *d*
5. *d*	**13.** *c*
6. *b*	**14.** *a*
7. *a*	**15.** *b*
8. *d*	

Analysis of Incorrect Answers

The correct answers to this quiz—the responses that best communicate acceptance and understanding—are those that characterize the correct responses. The *incorrect* answers can be characterized as fitting into the following four categories:

Directing: A response that tells or suggests to the message-sender what to do.

Warning: A response that warns the smoker what might happen.

Criticizing/disagreeing: A response that criticizes or disagrees with the smoker in that situation.

Diagnosing: A response that suggests an explanation for the message sender's statement.

	Directing	Warning	Criticizing/ Disagreeing	Diagnosing
1.	a		b	d
2.	c	d	a	
3.	b	c	a	
4.	c		d	b
5.	a		c	b
6.			d	a, c
7.	b	c	d	
8.	b	c	a	
9.	b	a	d	
10.	a, c			d
11.	d	c		b
12.	c		a, b	
13.		d	a	b
14.	d		b	c
15.	c		d	a

Quiz 5: Facts about Exercise

In this quiz, you will find statements about the effects of exercise. Some of the statements are true and some are false. Put your answer in the "True or False" column.

	True or False
1. People who are muscularly fit are automatically also cardiovascularly fit.	_____
2. Regular exercise increases the heart rate at rest.	_____
3. All the cardiovascular benefits that result from regular exercise are gradually lost if exercise is not continued.	_____
4. A single exercise session can have a lasting effect on the cardiovascular system.	_____
5. Muscles that are not exercised turn into fat.	_____
6. Regular exercise has no effect on the body's ability to use fat.	_____
7. Regular exercise combined with dieting is a more effective way to reduce fat than just dieting.	_____
8. The number of calories burned during exercise depends only on the type of exercise.	_____
9. A heavier person uses more calories than a lighter person.	_____
10. A person's physical fitness refers to how that person's body looks.	_____
11. Experts believe that there is no relationship between physical fitness and work performance.	_____
12. Exercise can provide an opportunity to make new friends.	_____

Answers

1.	F	**7.**	T
2.	F	**8.**	F
3.	T	**9.**	T
4.	F	**10.**	F
5.	F	**11.**	F
6.	F	**12.**	T

Quiz 6: Designing an Exercise Program

This test consists of questions about exercise program design. Some of the statements are true and some are false. Put your answer in the "True or False" column.

	True or False
1. Participating in an activity program where everyone exercises at the same level of intensity can be dangerous.	_____
2. An individual's exercise program does not need to specify the length of each exercise session.	_____
3. A conditioning program is used only for building muscular strength.	_____
4. The benefits gained from exercise depend, in part, on the number of days per week that a person exercises.	_____
5. The warm-up and stretching period of an exercise session should last from five to fifteen minutes.	_____
6. All individuals should see a doctor before starting an exercise program.	_____
7. An exercise program should include a cool-down period.	_____

	True or False
8. Warm-up and stretching exercises will have little effect on the muscle soreness a person often feels when first starting an exercise program.	_____
9. Cool-down activities help prevent soreness.	_____
10. The target level for a healthy person building cardiovascular endurance is 90 to 100 percent of one's maximum heart rate.	_____
11. Cardiovascular endurance refers to the ability of the body to perform rhythmical exercise for very short periods of time.	_____
12. Cardiovascular endurance activities must be repeated at least three times per week in order to get the most benefit.	_____
13. Swimming has little effect on one's cardiovascular endurance capacity.	_____
14. All sports provide the same benefits.	_____
15. Playing volleyball regularly improves one's cardiovascular endurance capacity.	_____
16. A regular exercise program does not need to take a great deal of time.	_____
17. Individuals exercising below their target heart rate show little improvement in cardiovascular fitness.	_____
18. Bicycling can improve one's cardiovascular endurance capacity.	_____

Answers

1. T	**4.** T
2. F	**5.** T
3. F	**6.** F

7. T	13. F
8. F	14. F
9. T	15. F
10. F	16. T
11. F	17. T
12. T	18. T

Quiz 7: Facts about Food

Not all the answers to questions in this quiz can be found in the book. Nonetheless, we thought the subject important enough to include even such questions. This test consists of twenty statements about food and nutrients. Some of the statements are true and some are false. Put your answer in the "True or False" columns.

	True or False
1. About 30 percent of a person's calorie intake should come from refined and processed sugars.	_____
2. A single food can supply all the nutrients that a person needs in order to meet the Recommended Dietary Allowances (RDA).	_____
3. Individuals get enough salt without adding salt to food when it is eaten.	_____
4. Saturated fats are fats which are usually obtained from plant sources—for example, corn.	_____
5. Saturated fats are usually solid at room temperature.	_____

	True or False
6. Raw fruits and vegetables have a high fiber content.	_____
7. A person who selects foods according to their nutrient content will be unable to plan a diet that meets the RDA standards.	_____
8. A person must eat a variety of foods in order to meet the RDA standards.	_____
9. Steaming foods such as vegetables prevents the loss of nutrients.	_____
10. The diets of most Americans are lacking in the necessary vitamins and minerals.	_____
11. Fruits contain complex carbohydrates.	_____
12. An extra amount of one nutrient will make up for a shortage of another nutrient.	_____
13. Alcohol can contribute many nutrients to a person's diet.	_____
14. About 50 percent of a person's recommended calorie intake should come from fats.	_____
15. Frying a food may destroy some of the nutrients found in that food.	_____
16. Naturally occurring sugars are sugars that are added to a food after it is grown.	_____
17. Honey is a food that has a low sugar content.	_____
18. The greater the variety of foods a person eats, the less risk there is of developing a deficiency of any one nutrient.	_____
19. Complex carbohydrates and naturally occurring sugars should make up about half (48 percent) of a person's recommended calorie intake.	_____
20. Foods which are baked increase in fat content.	_____

Answers

1. F	11. T
2. F	12. T
3. T	13. F
4. F	14. F
5. T	15. T
6. T	16. F
7. F	17. F
8. T	18. T
9. T	19. T
10. F	20. F

Quiz 8: Weight Management

This test consists of statements about weight management, an issue of vital importance to any new ex-smoker who is beginning to put on pounds. Some of the statements are true and some are false. Put your answer in the "True or False" column.

	True or False
1. An individual's percentage of total body fat decreases gradually with age.	_____
2. Excess body fat can contribute to the development of cardiovascular disease.	_____
3. Proteins supply calories.	_____
4. The goal of a reducing diet is to lower body weight by decreasing the amount of body fat.	_____
5. Weight loss will be the greatest during the first few weeks of a diet.	_____

	True or False
6. A reducing diet should contain all the nutrients recommended by the RDA.	_____
7. Flavored yogurt has a high sugar content.	_____
8. A healthy level of body fat for men is higher than it is for women.	_____
9. A weight-loss diet that permanently changes eating habits will have the least success.	_____
10. Calorie intake must drop below 800 calories a day before there is a risk of a diet lacking essential nutrients.	_____
11. Overweight individuals are often malnourished because they eat many low-nutrient, high-calorie foods.	_____
12. Body weight is determined by activity level and food consumption.	_____
13. Thinking requires a great deal of energy.	_____
14. Increasing the number of calories used (through exercise) and decreasing the number of calories eaten will usually result in weight loss.	_____
15. A person's age has no effect in determining that individual's calorie requirements.	_____
16. The body stores excess energy in the form of body fat.	_____
17. Creamed cottage cheese has a low fat content.	_____
18. When there is a balance between the total number of calories eaten and used, the intake of needed nutrients will also be adequate.	_____

Answers

1. F	**4.** T
2. T	**5.** T
3. T	**6.** T

7. T	**13.** F
8. F	**14.** T
9. F	**15.** F
10. F	**16.** T
11. T	**17.** F
12. T	**18.** F

Quiz 9: Making Diet Changes

The fictitious characters in this quiz all want to make certain changes in their eating habits. These individuals, however, want to make sure that they maintain a diet that provides all the recommended nutrients. In each case, circle the letter which is the best choice for the individual involved.

1. Hank wants to reduce the amount of salt in his diet. One appropriate way for Hank to do this is to:

    a. use seasonings such as catsup and soy sauce in place of salt.

    b. select products that list sodium nitrate or monosodium glutamate (MSG) as an ingredient.

    c. eat fresh foods rather than canned ones whenever possible.

    d. none of the above.

2. Grace wants to reduce the amount of fat in her diet. One appropriate way for Grace to do this is to:

    a. use margarine rather than butter for cooking and eating.

    b. eat more red meat and less chicken and fish.

    c. eat cheese or nuts for snacks instead of potato chips or doughnuts.

    d. none of the above.

3. Sue wants to reduce the number of calories in her diet. One appropriate way for Sue to do this is to:

    a. substitute fish for meat whenever possible.

    b. eat flavored gelatin rather than ice cream for dessert.

    c. eat whole-grain rather than white bread products.

    d. none of the above.

4. Mel wants to increase the amount of fiber in his diet. One appropriate way for Mel to do this is to:

    a. select bread products that are labeled "enriched" or "fortified."

    b. eat more raw fruits and vegetables.

    c. eat more cheese and yogurt.

    d. none of the above.

5. Harriet wants to reduce the amount of sugar in her diet. One appropriate way for Harriet to do this is to:

    a. look for products that list "sucrose" or "dextrose" rather than sugar as an ingredient.

    b. eat ice milk instead of ice cream.

    c. select fruits canned in their own juice rather than in syrup.

    d. none of the above.

6. Carol wants to reduce the number of calories in her diet. One appropriate way for Carol to do this is to:

    a. drink nonfat rather than whole milk.

    b. select products that indicate they contain only natural ingredients.

    c. cook with a shortening that is liquid rather than solid at room temperature.

    d. none of the above.

7. Arthur wants to reduce the amount of fat in his diet. One appropriate way for Arthur to do this is to:

    a. use meat drippings rather than gravy to season his meat.

    b. select products made with coconut oil rather than shortening.

    c. limit the amount of baked goods such as cookies and pies that he eats.

    d. none of the above.

8. Diane wants to reduce the number of calories in her diet. One appropriate way for Diane to do this is to:

   a. season vegetables with butter or margarine rather than with cream sauces.

   b. eat most of her fruits and vegetables raw rather than cooked.

   c. eliminate most dairy products from her diet.

   d. none of the above.

Answers

1. *c*	**5.** *c*
2. *d*	**6.** *a*
3. *a*	**7.** *c*
4. *b*	**8.** *d*

SURVIVAL TECHNIQUES: A CAPSULE GUIDE FOR THE NEW EX-SMOKER

There are times when it may be a bit inconvenient to carry this book around with you. Yet it is important to keep it handy for review and reference should you encounter a crisis situation pertaining to smoking.

The following guide is a capsulized review of the important points outlined in the pages of this book. You may want to run these few pages through a duplicating machine and tuck them into your purse or wallet or simply keep them in your desk drawer at work. They will serve as a refresher course for you, reinforcing important survival techniques you have learned through a careful reading of this guide.

Body Language: The ABCs of Withdrawal

1. Expect a variety of symptoms and sensations upon quitting smoking, such as tingling sensations, some dizziness, nervousness, irritation, and other mood swings. Don't panic. Such withdrawal symptoms will disappear or diminish considerably within four weeks.

2. Try to keep track of your mood changes by keeping a record of them in a chart like the one shown in the book. It is an important first step in dealing with such mood swings.

The Body Eclectic

1. Beware of emotional "triggers" that may tempt you to reach for a cigarette. Boredom, stress—even happiness—can make you want to light up. Physical triggers can be such things as watching television or the end of a meal.

2. If you are now substituting food for cigarettes, you are likely to develop a weight problem. You must remain aware of this happening. Keep a record of your eating habits for at least a week, using a chart like the one shown in the book.

The Double Whammy

1. The amount and kind of physical activity you engage in can tip the scale to either thin or fat. Even moderate physical activity burns off unwanted calories.

2. Exercise is the key that unlocks every door to weight control, so get going on some kind of regular program.

3. The best kind of physical activity for both fitness and weight control should include some form of aerobic exercise. Swimming, cycling, jogging, and walking are some examples. Choose a fun exercise that will keep you going nonstop from fifteen to forty minutes each day. A lunch-hour walk is perfect.

4. Pay attention to your heart rate during exercise. Make sure it is beating at between 60 and 75 percent of your maximum heart rate during exercise.

Even Ex-Smokers Get the Blues

Feeling depressed after you quit smoking is a normal reaction to the withdrawal process. You are not going crazy, so don't call a therapist! Exercise will give a tremendous boost to your sagging spirits.

How Do You Spell Relief?

1. Exercise not only helps ward off the blues and other negative withdrawal symptoms caused by the absence of nicotine, but is also one of the best tools for weight control.

2. Avoid boring situations. Try to keep busy or active. Join a club, find a new hobby, go out and dance. Maybe even think about a new job if this one is tempting you to smoke.

3. Feeling angry? Or depressed? Deep breathing may be the solution. Try the following exercise and watch your mood change:

   a. With your mouth closed and shoulders relaxed, inhale as slowly and deeply as you can while silently counting to eight. As you're doing this, push your stomach out.

b. Hold that breath to the count of four.

c. Exhale slowly, again to the count of eight.

d. Repeat this inhale/exhale cycle five times.

4. Do you have a sudden craving for a cigarette? Practice the straw exercise or chew on a raw carrot. All such exercises are designed to play on time until the urge passes.

You Are What You Eat

1. Avoid snacks. If you must nibble, try fruits or nuts.

2. For the first few weeks of not smoking, avoid meat, sugar, alcohol, cheese, and eggs.

3. Eat less, more slowly. Make a meal last at least twenty minutes.

4. Increase your physical activity at home and at the office. Walk when you usually drive. Stand when you can sit, etc.

Food for Thought

1. Involve family and friends in your effort to remain smokeless.

2. Be pleasant but firm with relatives or friends who want to treat you with gifts of food.

3. Pay attention not only to the type and amount of food you eat, but also to how the food you eat is cooked. Try to eat only foods that are broiled, baked, steamed, or boiled, with the fat trimmed away before cooking.

4. Avoid cream, butter, and sauces. Drink sugar-free beverages.

5. Be patient with your weight-loss program. Be realistic. Don't set your goals too high. A loss of one to two pounds a week is a success story. Remember: Small changes eventually lead to greater changes.

A Pocket Full of Miracles

1. Avoid fad diets.
2. Make sure any reducing diet you try is nutritionally sound.
3. The best diet plan is a well-balanced one. So eat a variety of foods.
4. Try to eat less fat and more carbohydrates. Avoid saturated fats in your diet.
5. Diets containing less than 800 calories may be hazardous to your health.

If at First You Don't Succeed

Remember! If you do sneak a smoke it is not the end of the world. Don't let this one slip-up defeat your goal to be a non-smoker. Pick up where you left off.

Say It Again, Sam

If someone teases you about not smoking or tries to pressure you into having just one, assert yourself! Calmly express your feelings and stand up for your rights. Don't get angry and don't run from such a situation. Deal with it in a manner that maintains your self-respect and creates little tension.

Visualization: To Be or Not to Be

You may have a tense situation with the boss coming up, or a speech to make in front of 200 people. Don't reach for a cigarette, but for your imagination, instead. Take a few minutes to visualize yourself in such situations. See yourself as calm and successful and you will be! Use this technique in any pressure situation—business, social, or other.

One Is the Loneliest Number

Giving up cigarettes can, at times, be a tough, lonely road. Why travel it by yourself? Get involved in a support group or, if there isn't any in your area, why not form one of your own?

HELP FROM ORGANIZATIONS AND AGENCIES

For answers to questions about smoking cessation, general information on smoking, free literature, or referrals to local services, you may write or call the following organizations and agencies:

Action on Smoking and Health
2000 H Street NW
Washington, DC 20006
202-659-4310

American Cancer Society
777 Third Avenue
New York, New York 10017
212-371-2900

American Health Foundation
Department of Behavioral Sciences
1370 Avenue of the Americas
New York, New York 10019
212-489-8700

American Heart Association
7320 Greenville Avenue
Dallas, Texas 75231
214-750-5300

American Lung Association
1740 Broadway
New York, New York 10019
212-315-8700

Canadian Council on Smoking and Health
3430 O'Connor
Ottawa, Ontario K2P1V9
613-236-6035

Cancer Information Clearinghouse
7910 Woodmont Avenue
Suite 1320
Bethesda, Maryland 20014
301-565-5955

National Association on Smoking and Health
4155 East Jewel Avenue
Denver, Colorado 80237
303-753-0777

National Cancer Institute
National Institutes of Health
Bethesda, Maryland 20014
301-496-6641

National Clearinghouse for Smoking and Health
Atlanta, Georgia 30333
404-633-3311

National Heart, Lung and Blood Institute
National Institutes of Health
Bethesda, Maryland 20205
301-496-4236

National Interagency Council on Smoking and Health
419 Park Avenue South
New York, New York 10016
212-532-6035

Office on Smoking and Health
Department of Health and Human Services
5600 Fishers Lane
Rockville, Maryland 20857
301-443-1575

SmokEnders
Memorial Parkway
Phillipsburg, New Jersey 08865
201-454-HELP

The Tobacco Institute
1776 K Street NW
Washington, DC 20006
202-457-4800

The Cancer Information Service

The Cancer Information Service, sponsored by the US Public Health Service, is a toll-free telephone inquiry system that supplies information about smoking to the general public. It also provides free printed materials on the subject. You can reach the service by dialing the number for your state listed below:

Alabama: 1-800-292-6201

Alaska: 1-800-638-6070

California: 1-800-252-9066 (from area codes 213, 714, and 805 only)

Colorado: 1-800-332-1850

Connecticut: 1-800-922-0824

Delaware: 1-800-523-3586

District of Columbia: 636-5700

Florida: 1-800-432-5953

Georgia: 1-800-327-7332

Hawaii: 808-524-1234 (on Oahu; from neighbor islands, call collect)

Illinois: 1-800-972-0586

Kentucky: 1-800-432-9321

Maine: 1-800-225-7034

Maryland: 1-800-492-1444

Massachusetts: 1-800-952-7420

Michigan: 1-800-482-4959

Minnesota: 1-800-582-5262

New Hampshire: 1-800-225-7034

New Jersey: 1-800-223-1000 (northern); 1-800-523-3586 (southern)

New York: 1-800-462-7255; 212-794-7982 (in New York City)

North Carolina: 1-800-672-0943

North Dakota: 1-800-328-5188

Ohio: 1-800-282-6522

Pennsylvania: 1-800-822-3963

South Dakota: 1-800-328-5188

Texas: 1-800-392-2040

Vermont: 1-800-225-7034

Washington: 1-800-552-7212

Wisconsin: 1-800-362-8038

For all other states: 1-800-638-6694

Available Materials

Free or low-cost materials on all aspects of smoking and giving up cigarettes are available from a variety of agencies across the country. Here are a sampling of some of those materials. For more information, write or call the listed agencies.

Printed Matter

Eight Reasons Young People Smoke. National Clearinghouse for Smoking and Health.

No Smoking, Lungs at Work. American Lung Association.

As You Live . . . You Breathe. American Lung Association.

Huff 'n Puff. American Cancer Society.

Surprising News about Women. National Clearinghouse for Smoking and Health.

Women Are Kicking the Habit. American Lung Association.

When a Woman Smokes. American Cancer Society.

Cigarette Smoking. American Lung Association.

If You Must Smoke (information on tar and nicotine content). National Clearinghouse for Smoking and Health.

Facts: Smoking and Health.   National Clearinghouse for Smoking and Health.

Be Kind to Nonsmokers.   American Lung Association.

Second Hand Smoke.   American Lung Association.

If You Want to Give Up Cigarettes.   American Cancer Society.

Remember When?   American Lung Association.

Q&A of Smoking and Health.   American Lung Association

Cigarette Quiz.   American Heart Association.

What Everyone Should Know about Smoking and Heart Disease.   American Heart Association.

Slim and Smokeless.   National Clearinghouse on Smoking and Health.

Films

Everything You Always Wanted to Know about How to Stop Smoking but Were Afraid to Ask.   American Lung Association.

Is It Worth Your Life.   American Lung Association.

Point of View (teens and adults).   American Lung Association.

The Benefits of Quitting Smoking.   American Cancer Society.

Health Aspects of Quitting.   American Cancer Society.

Insights into the Quitting Process.   American Cancer Society.

Helping and Being Helped.   American Cancer Society

Posters

"Thank You for Not Smoking."   American Lung Association & American Heart Association.

"We All Share the Same Air."   American Lung Association.

"Lungs at Work, No Smoking" (also in tentcards and buttons).   American Lung Association.

BIBLIOGRAPHY

A Special Introduction: For Smokers Only

American Lung Association. *Freedom from Smoking in 20 Days: A Self-Help Quit Smoking Program from the American Lung Association.* New York: American Lung Association, 1980.

US Department of Health and Human Services. *A Self-Test for Smokers.* Washington, DC: Government Printing Office, 1980.

US Department of Health and Human Services (Public Health Service and National Institutes of Health). *Clearing the Air: A Guide to Quitting Smoking. Washington DC: Government Printing Office, 1984.*

Body Language: The ABC's of Withdrawal

Gilbert, M., and Pope, Marilyn A. "Effects of Quitting Smoking." *Psychopharmacology* 78 (1982): 121–127.

Shiffman, Saul M., and Jarvik, Murray E. "Smoking Withdrawal

Symptoms in Two Weeks of Abstinence." *Psychopharmacology* 50 (1976): 35–39.

Wynder, Ernest L.; Kaufman, Paul L.; and Lesser, Robert L. "A Short-Term Followup Study on Ex-Cigarette Smokers." *American Review of Respiratory Diseases,* 1967.

Smoke Gets in Your Eyes

Balfour, D. J. K. "The Pharmacology of Nicotine Dependence: A Working Hypothesis." *Pharmacology and Therapeutics* 15 (1982): 239–250.

Gonzalez, Elizabeth R. "Snuffing Out the Cigarette Habit: How About Another Source of Nicotine?" *JAMA* 244, no. 2 (July 10, 1980): 112–113.

Isaac, P., and Rand, M. "Cigarette Smoking and Plasma Levels of Nicotine." *Nature* 236 (1972): 308–310.

Pomerleau, Ovide F. "Underlying Mechanisms in Substance Abuse: Examples from Research on Smoking." *Addictive Behaviors* 6 (1981): 187–196.

Pomerleau, Ovide F.; Fertig, Joanne B.; and Shanahan, Sandra O. "Nicotine Dependence in Cigarette Smoking: An Empirically-Based, Multivariate Model." *Pharmacology Biochemistry and Behavior* 19 (1983): 291–299.

The Second World Conference on Smoking and Health. London: Washington, DC: Government Printing Office, 1972.

US Department of Health and Human Services. *Smoking and Health.* Washington, DC: Government Printing Office, 1983.

US Department of Health, Education and Welfare. *Adult Use of Tobacco.* Washington, DC: Government Printing Office, 1975.

US Surgeon General's Report and National Center for Health Statistics. *Cigarette Smoking and Health.* Washington, DC: Government Printing Office, 1979.

Work Group 1 of the World Conference on Smoking and Health. "Addiction, Habituation and Pharmacology of Tobacco." *Summary of the Proceedings of the World Conference on Smoking and Health.* Washington, DC: Government Printing Office, 1976.

The Body Eclectic

Bosse, R.; Garvey, A. J.; and Costa, A. T. "Weight Change Following Smoking Cessation." *International Journal of Addictions* 15 (1980): 983–988.

Brozek, J., and Keys, A. "Changes of Body Weight in Normal Men Who Stop Smoking Cigarettes." *Science,* June 14, 1957, p. 1203.

Glauser, Elinor M.; Reidenberg, Marcus M.; Rusy, Ben F.; and Tallarida, Ronald J. "Study Explains Post-Smokers' Pounds." *JAMA* 209, no. 11 (September 15, 1969): 1621–1622.

Gordon, Tavia; Kannel, William B.; Dawber, Thomas R.; and McGee, Daniel. "Changes Associated with Quitting Cigarette Smoking: The Framington Study." *American Heart Journal* 90 (September 1975): 322–328.

Grunberg, Neil E. "The Effects of Nicotine and Cigarette Smoking on Food Consumption and Taste Preferences." *Addictive Behaviors* 7 (1982): 317–331.

Lincoln, Jetson E. "Weight Gain after Cessation of Smoking." To the Editor. *JAMA* 210, no. 9 (December 1, 1969): 1765.

Noppa, Henry, and Bengtsson, Calle. "Obesity in Relation to Smoking: A Population Study of Women in Goteborg, Sweden." *Preventive Medicine* 9 (1980): 534–543.

Wack, Jeffery T., and Rodin, Judith. "Smoking and Its Effects on Body Weight and the Systems of Caloric Regulation. *American Journal of Clinical Nutrition,* February 1982, pp. 366–380.

The Double Whammy

American College of Sports Medicine. "The Recommended Quantity and Quality of Exercise for Developing and Maintaining Fitness in Healthy Adults." *Medicine and Science* 10 (1978): 219–225.

American Medical Association. "Research on the Riddle of Obesity Gains New Scientific Weight." *JAMA* 239 (1982): 1727–1732.

Bahrke, M. S., and Morgan, W. P. "Anxiety Reduction Following Exercise and Meditation." *Cognitive Therapy and Research* 2 (1978): 323–333.

Bjorntorp, B. "Exercise in the Treatment of Obesity." *Clinics in Endocrinology and Metabolism* 5 (1976): 431–453.

Epstein, Leonard H., and Wing, Rena R. "Aerobic Exercise and Weight." *Addictive Behaviors* 5 (1980): 371–378.

President's Council on Physical Fitness and Sports. *Exercise and Weight Control.* Washington, DC: Government Printing Office, 1980.

———. *Fitness Fundamentals.* Washington, DC: Government Printing Office, 1984.

Thompson, J. Keven; Jarvie, J. Gregory; and Lahey, B. Benjamin. "Etiology, Physiology and Intervention." *Psychological Bulletin* 91, no. 1 (1982): 55–79.

These Boots Are Made for Walking

Lion, Lionel S. "Psychological Effects of Jogging: A Preliminary Study." *Perceptual and Motor Skills* 47 (1978): 1215–1218.

President's Council on Physical Fitness and Sports. *An Introduction to Physical Fitness.* Washington, DC: Government Printing Office, 1984.

———. *Aqua Dynamics: Water Exercises Are the New Way to Stay in Shape.* Washington, DC: Government Printing Office, 1983.

———. *Exercise and Your Heart.* Washington, DC: Government Printing Office, 1984.

———. *One Step At a Time.* Washington, DC: Government Printing Office, 1984.

———. *Swimming and Bicycling.* Washington, DC: Government Printing Office, 1977.

US Department of Health and Human Services, Public Health Service and National Institutes of Health. *Exercise and Your Heart.* Washington, DC: Government Printing Office, 1981.

Even Ex-Smokers Get the Blues

Chernick, V. "The Brain's Own Morphine and Cigarette Smoking: The Junkie in Disguise?" *Chest,* January 1983, pp. 2–4.

Cryer, Phillip E.; Haymond, Morey W.; Santiago, Julio V.; and Shah, Suresh D. "Norepinephrine and Epinephrine Release and Adrenergic Mediation of Smoking-Associated Hemodynamic and Metabolic Events." *New England Journal of Medicine* 295 (September 9, 1976): 573–577.

Hill, Peter, and Wynder, Ernest L. "Smoking and Cardiovascular Disease." *American Heart Journal* 87, no. 4 (April 1974): 491–496.

Kline, Nathan S., and Lehmann, Heinz E. "Clinical Observations with Beta-Endorphin Injections." *Psychopharmacology Bulletin* 14, no. 3 (1978): 12–13.

Kline, Nathan S.; Li, Choh Houo; Lehmann, Heinz E.; Lajtha, Abel; Laski, Edward; and Cooper, Tomas. "B-Endorphin Induced Changes in Schizophrenic and Depressed Patients." *Archives of General Psychiatry* 34 (September 1977): 1111–1113.

McGeer, P. L., and McGeer, E. G. "Chemistry of Mood and Emotion." *Annual Review Psychological,* 1980, pp. 273–307.

Pomerleau, Ovide F.; Fertig, Joanne B.; Fertig, L.; Seyler, Everett; and Jaffe, Jerome. "Neuroendocrine Reactivity to Nicotine in Smokers." *Psychopharmacology* 81 (1983): 61–67.

Prince, Raymond. "The Endorphins: A Review for Psychological Anthropologists." *Ethos* 10, no. 4 (Winter 1982): 303–316.

Risch, Samuel C., and Cohen, Robert M. "Mood and Behavioral Effects of Physostigmine on Humans Are Accompanied by Elevations in Plasma B-Endorphin and Cortisol." *Science* 209 (September 1980): 1545–1546.

Scarf, Maggie. *Unfinished Business: Pressure Points in the Lives of Women.* New York: Ballantine Books, 1981.

How Do You Spell Relief?

Appenzeller, Otto; Standefer, Jim; Appenzeller, Judith; and Atkinson, Ruth. "Neurology of Endurance Training V. Endorphins." *Neurology* 30 (April 1980): 418–419.

Barchas, Jack David, and Berger, Phillip A. "Endogenous Opiods: Basic and Clinical Aspects." *Psychopharmacology Bulletin* 16 (1980): 51–52.

Beary, John F., and Benson, Herbert. "A Simple Psychophysiologic Technique Which Elicits the Hypometabolic Changes of the Relaxation Response." *Psychosomatic Medicine* 36, no. 2 (March-April 1974): 115–117.

Benson, Herbert. "The Relaxation Response: Its Subjective and Objective Historical Precedents and Physiology." *Trends in Neurosciences,* July 1983, pp. 281–284.

Benson, Herbert; Arns, Patricia A.; and Hoffman, John W. "The Relaxation Response and Hypnosis." *International Journal of Clinical and Experimental Hypnosis* 29, no. 3 (1981): 259–270.

Berger, Bonnie G., and Owen, David R. "Mood Alteration with Swimming—Swimmers Really Do 'Feel Better.'" *Psychosomatic Medicine* 45 (October 1983): 425–431.

Blue, Richard F. "Aerobic Running as a Treatment for Moderate Depression." *Perceptual and Motor Skills* 48 (1979): 28.

Boswell, Philip C., and Murray, Edward J. "Effects of Meditation on Psychological and Physiological Measures of Anxiety." *Journal of Consulting and Clinical Psychology* 47, no. 3 (1979): 606–607.

Carr, Daniel B.; Bullen, Beverly A.; Skrinar, Gary S.; Arnold, Michael A.; Rosenblatt, Michael; Beitins, Inesez; Martin, Joseph B.; and McArthur, Janet. "Physical Conditioning Facilitates the Exercise-Induced Secretion of Beta-Endorphin and Beta-Lipotropin in Women." *New England Journal of Medicine* 305, no. 10 (September 3, 1981): 560–563.

Colt, Edward W. D.; Wardlaw, Sharon; and Frantz, Andrew G. "The Effect of Running on Plasma B-Endorphin." *Life Sciences* 28 (1981): 1637–1640.

Emrich, H. M., and Millan, M. J. "Stress Reactions and Endorphinergic Systems. *Journal of Psychosomatic Research* 26, no. 2 (1982): 101–104.

Farrell, Peter A.; Gates, Ward K.; Maksod, Michael G.; and Morgan, William P. "Increases in Plasma B-Endorphin/B-Lipotropin Immunoreactivity after Treadmill Running in Humans." *Journal of Applied Physiology* 52, no. 5 (1982): 1245–1249.

Fraioli, F. C.; Moretti, C.; Paolucci, D.; Alicicco, E.; Crescenzi, F.; and Fortunio, G. "Physical Exercise Stimulates Marked Concomitant Release of B-Endorphin and Adrenocorticotropic Hormone (ACTH) in Peripheral Blood in Man." *Experientia* 36 (1980): 987–989.

Fuller, John A. "Smoking Withdrawal and Acupuncture." *Medical Journal of Australia,* January 9, 1982, pp. 28–29.

Gondola, Joan C., and Tuckman, Bruce W. "Effect of Training and Mood Enhancement in Women Runners." *Perceptual and Motor Skills* 57 (1983): 333–334.

Greist, John H.; Klein, Marjorie H.; Eischens, Roger R.; Faris, John; Gurman, Alan S.; and Morgan, William P. "Running as a Treatment for Depression." *Comprehensive Psychiatry* 20, no. 1 (1979): 41–53.

Gwynne, Peter. "Acupuncture Update." *Todays Health,* January 1974, p. 16.

Harber, Victoria J., and Sutton, John R. "Endorphins and Exercise." *Sports Medicine* 1 (1984): 154–171.

Harvey, John R. "The Effect of Yogic Breathing Exercises on Mood." *Journal of the American Society of Psychosomatic Dentistry and Medicine* 30, no. 2 (1983): 39–48.

Harvey, John R. "A Practical Technique for Breath Control." *Behavior Therapist* 1, no. 2 (1978): 13–15.

Janal, Malvin N.; Colt, Edward W. D.; Clark, W. Crawford; and Glusman, Murray. "Pain Sensitivity, Mood and Plasma Endocrine Levels in Man Following Long Distance Running: Effects of Naloxone." *Pain* 19 (1984): 13–25.

Levi, Lennart. "The Urinary Output of Adrenalin and Noradrenalin During Pleasant and Unpleasant Emotional States." *Psychosomatic Medicine* 27 (1965): 80–85.

Lion, Lionel S. "Psychological Effects of Jogging: A Preliminary Study." *Perceptual and Motor Skills* 47 (1978): 1215–1218.

MacHovec, Frank J., and Man, S. C. "Acupuncture and Hypnosis Compared: Fifty-eight Cases." *American Journal of Clinical Hypnosis* 21 (July 1978): 45–47.

Martin, G. P., and Waite, P. M. E. "The Efficacy of Acupuncture as an Aid to Stopping Smoking." *New Zealand Medical Journal,* June 24, 1981, 421–423.

Martin, Rod A., and Lefcourt, Herbert M. "Sense of Humor as a Moderator of the Relation Between Stressors and Moods." *Journal of Personality and Social Psychology* 45 (1983): 1313–1324.

Michaels, R. R.; Huber, M. J.; and McCann, D. S. "Evaluation of Transcendental Meditation as a Method of Reducing Stress." *Science* 192 (1976): 1242–1244.

Morgan, William F. "Anxiety Reduction Following Acute Physical Activity." *Psychiatric Annals,* March 1979, 36–45.

Paul, Gordon L. "Physiological Effects of Relaxation Training and Hypnotic Suggestion." *Journal of Abnormal Psychology* 74, no. 4 (1969): 425–437.

Pomeranz, Bruce. "Acupuncture and the Endorphins." *Ethos* 10, no. 4 (Winter 1982): 385–393.

Pomeranz, Bruce, and Chiu, Daryl. "Naloxone Blockage of Acupuncture Analgesia: Endorphin Implicated." *Life Sciences* 19 (1976): 1757–1762.

Smith, Philip. *Total Breathing.* New York: McGraw-Hill, 1980, p. 54.

Speads, Carola H. *Breathing: The ABC's.* New York: Harper and Row, 1978, pp. 44, 116.

Suinn, R., and Richardson, F. "Anxiety Management Training: A Non-Specific Behavior Therapy Program for Anxiety Control." *Behavior Therapy* 2 (1971): 498–510.

Wallace, Robert Keith, and Benson, Herbert. "The Physiology of Meditation." *Scientific American,* 1972, pp. 85–90.

West, Michael A. "Physiological Effects of Meditation: A Longitudinal Study." *British Journal of Social and Clinical Psychology* 18 (1979): 219–226.

Wilson, V. E.; Morley, N. C.; and Bird, E. I. "Mood Profiles of Marathon Runners, Joggers and Non-Exercisers." *Perceptual and Motor Skills* 50 (1980): 117–118.

You Are What You Eat (I)

American Dietetic Association and US Department of Agriculture. *Food 2.* 1982.

Breithaupt, Sandra, and Agnew, Wayne H. *The Dallas Doctor's Diet.* New York: McGraw-Hill, 1983.

"How to Stay Slender for Life." *Reader's Digest,* October 1982. Condensed from *Executive Health,* March 1982, Executive Health Publications, P.O. Box 589, Rancho Santa Fe, Calif. 92067.

Levitz, S. "Behavioral Therapy in Treating Obesity." *Journal of the American Dietetic Association* 62 (1973): 22–26.

You Are What You Eat (II)

American Dietetic Association and US Department of Agriculture. *Food 2.* 1982.

Fields, Frank. *Take It Off with Frank.* New York: William Morrow, 1977.

Katch, Frank J. *Nutrition, Weight Control and Exercise.* Boston: Houghton Mifflin, 1977.

Mandell, Marshall, and Gare, Fran. *It's Not Your Fault You're Fat Diet.* New York: Harper & Row, 1983.

Williams, Sue Rodwell. *Nutrition and Diet Therapy.* St. Louis: C. V. Mosby, 1977.

Food for Thought

Gibson, H. B. "A Form of Behavior Therapy for Some States Diagnosed as 'Affective Disorder.' " *Behavioral, Respiratory Therapy* 16 (1978): 191–195.

Grinstead, O. A. "A Comparison of Behavioral Treatment Approaches." PhD dissertation, University of California at Los Angeles, 1981.

Levitz, Leonard S. "Behavior Therapy in Treating Obesity." *Journal of the American Dietetic Association* 62 (January 1973).

Stollack, George. "Weight Loss Obtained under Different Experimental Procedures." *Psychotherapy* 4 (1967): 61–67.

Stunkard, Alan J. "New Therapies for the Eating Disorders: Behavior Modification of Obesity and Anorexia Nervosa." *Archives of General Psychiatry* 76 (1972): 391–400.

A Pocket Full of Miracles

American Dietetic Association and US Department of Agriculture. *Food 2.* 1982.

Berland, Theodore. *Consumer Guide's Rating the Diets.* Chicago: Rand McNally, 1982.

Chicago Heart Association. *The Heart Saver Eating Guide.* 1982.

Department of Health, Bureau of Nutrition, New York City. *Count Your Calories.* 1974.

————. *Eat to Lose Weight.* 1983.

US Department of Agriculture. *Nutrition and Your Health.* Washington, DC: Government Printing Office, 1980.

If at First You Don't Succeed . . .

Eisinger, Richard A. "Psychosocial Predictors of Smoking Recidivism." *Journal of Health and Social Behavior* 12 (December 1971): 355–358.

Schacter, Stanley. "Recidivism and Self-Cure of Smoking and Obesity." *American Psychologist* 37 (April 1982): 436–444.

Shiffman, Saul. "Relapse Following Smoking Cessation: A Situational Analysis." *Journal of Consulting and Clinical Psychology* 50 (1982): 71–86.

Say It Again, Sam

Baer, Jean. *How to Be an Assertive (Not Aggressive) Woman in Life, in Love, and on the Job.* New York: New American Library, 1976.

Smith, Manuel J. *When I Say No, I Feel Guilty.* New York: Bantam Books, 1975.

Visualization: To Be or Not to Be

Notes from a course on DMA by Robert Fritz.

One Is the Loneliest Number

Bates, Richard C. "Let Problem Patients Help Each Other." *Medical Economist* 10 (July 1967) 124–136.

New York City Self-Help Clearinghouse. *How to Organize a Self-Help Group.* 1979. A publication of the New York City Self-Help Clearinghouse and the Graduate School and University Center of The City University of New York.

US Department of Health and Human Services. *Plain Talk about Mutual Help Groups.* Washington, DC: Government Printing Office, 1981.

INDEX